Obesity Prevention and Treatment

Lifestyle Medicine

Series Editor

James M. Rippe

Founder and Director, Rippe Lifestyle Institute
Professor of Medicine, University of Massachusetts Medical School

Led by James M. Rippe, MD, Founder and Director, Rippe Lifestyle Institute, this series is directed to a broad range of researchers and professionals consisting of topical books with clinical applications in nutrition and health, physical activity, obesity management, and applicable subjects in lifestyle medicine.

Increasing Physical Activity
A Practical Guide
James M. Rippe

Manual of Lifestyle Medicine
James M. Rippe

Obesity Prevention and Treatment
A Practical Guide
James M. Rippe and John P. Foreyt

For more information, please visit: www.routledge.com/Lifestyle-Medicine/book-series/CRCLM

Obesity Prevention and Treatment
A Practical Guide

Edited by
James M. Rippe, MD
Founder and Director, Rippe Lifestyle Institute
Professor of Medicine, University of
Massachusetts Medical School

John P. Foreyt, PhD
Professor, Department of Medicine, Baylor College of Medicine

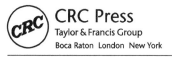

CRC Press
Taylor & Francis Group
Boca Raton London New York

CRC Press is an imprint of the
Taylor & Francis Group, an **informa** business

First edition published 2022
by CRC Press
6000 Broken Sound Parkway NW, Suite 300, Boca Raton, FL 33487-2742

and by CRC Press
2 Park Square, Milton Park, Abingdon, Oxon, OX14 4RN

Library of Congress Cataloging-in-Publication Data
Names: Rippe, James M., editor. | Foreyt, John Paul, editor.
Title: Obesity prevention and treatment : a practical guide / edited by James M. Rippe, John P. Foreyt.
Description: Boca Raton : CRC Press, 2022. | Includes bibliographical references and index. | Summary: "The World Health Organization estimates that there are 2.1 billion individuals with obesity globally. Nearly three quarters of adults in the United States are overweight or obese. The average individual with obesity cuts ten years off their life expectancy, yet less than 40% of physicians routinely counsel individuals concerning the adverse health consequences of obesity. Obesity Prevention and Treatment: A Practical Guide equips healthcare practitioners to include effective weight management counselling in the daily practice of medicine. Written by lifestyle medicine pioneer and cardiologist, Dr. James Rippe and obesity expert Dr. John Foreyt, this book provides evidence-based discussions of obesity and its metabolic consequences. A volume in the Lifestyle Medicine Series, it provides evidence-based information about the prevention and treatment of obesity through lifestyle measures, such as regular physical activity and sound nutrition, as well as the use of new medications or bariatric surgery available to assist in weight management. Provides a framework and practical strategies to assist practitioners in safe and effective treatments of obesity. Contains information explaining the relationship between obesity and increased risk of heart disease, diabetes, cancer, osteoarthritis, and other chronic conditions. Chapters begin with bulleted key points and conclude with a list of Clinical Applications. Written for practitioners at all levels, this user-friendly, evidence-based book on obesity prevention and treatment will be valuable to practitioners in general medicine or subspecialty practices"— Provided by publisher.
Identifiers: LCCN 2021017357 (print) | LCCN 2021017358 (ebook) |
ISBN 9780367551780 (paperback) | ISBN 9780367567187 (hardback) | ISBN 9781003099116 (ebook)
Subjects: MESH: Obesity—prevention & control | Obesity—therapy | Obesity—complications | United States
Classification: LCC RC628 (print) | LCC RC628 (ebook) | NLM QU 248 AA1 | DDC 616.3/98—dc23
LC record available at https://lccn.loc.gov/2021017357
LC ebook record available at https://lccn.loc.gov/2021017358

ISBN: 9780367567187 (hbk)
ISBN: 9780367551780 (pbk)
ISBN: 9781003099116 (ebk)

DOI: 10.1201/9781003099116

Typeset in Times
by codeMantra

Dedication

To my family, Stephanie, Hart, Jaelin, Devon and Jamie Rippe. Their love and support make all of these endeavors possible and worthwhile.

In memory of Julian Davis and Sam Cunningham, two of Dr. Foreyt's earliest clinical mentors, who both recently passed away, at ages 99 and 96, respectively, for their lifelong friendship. They will always be in my thoughts and prayers.

Contents

SECTION I   The Modern Management of Obesity

SECTION II   Obesity and Specific Medical Conditions

SECTION III   Future Directions and Public Health Issues

Preface

Obesity is a worldwide pandemic representing one of the most significant global public health issues. It is currently estimated that 2.1 billion people in the world are obese. Obesity significantly contributes to both worldwide morbidity and mortality.

In 2013, obesity was recognized by the American Medical Association as a disease. There is abundant research that supports that obesity increases the risk of many chronic diseases including cardiovascular disease (CVD), type 2 diabetes (T2DM), cancer, chronic kidney disease, and many musculoskeletal disorders. In the United States, both overweight and obesity are extremely common. The prevalence of obesity in the United States is estimated at 42.5%, while more than 73% of the population is considered overweight or obese. The prevalence of obesity has increased dramatically in the United States in the past 30–40 years. This has been attributed to increased consumption of calorie-dense foods as well as decreased level of physical activity.

Given the high prevalence of overweight and obesity, there is an urgent need to discover and promote effective treatments for both conditions. Furthermore, strategies to minimize weight gain which may contribute to lowering the prevalence of overweight and obesity are also very important.

Since both overweight and obesity carry significant adverse medical implications, it is incumbent upon healthcare professionals to be knowledgeable about both the treatment and prevention of these conditions. Moreover, since even small amounts of weight gain increase the risk of a variety of chronic conditions, strategies to prevent weight gain, even in healthy weight individuals, are very important.

Sadly, the medical profession has not been as active as we should have been in the prevention and treatment of overweight and obesity. It has been estimated that less than 40% of overweight or obese individuals are counseled concerning these conditions by their physician. This represents a significant wasted opportunity since more than 70% of individuals see their primary care physician on at least an annual basis.

Habits and practices that individuals can maintain in their daily lives carry enormous implications for lowering the risk of both overweight and obesity. Both physical activity and proper nutrition play crucial roles in weight loss, reducing weight gain and maintaining healthy body weight. These two modalities are also central to the emerging field of lifestyle medicine.

This book, *Obesity Prevention and Treatment: A Practical Guide*, will cover a variety of important areas related to the modern understandings and management of obesity. Specifically, emphasized will be how such daily lifestyle habits and actions such as regular physical activity and proper nutrition contribute not only to lowering the risk of weight gain and obesity but also lower the risk of comorbidities such as CVD, T2DM, and cancer.

While it may seem simple that either decreased caloric intake or increased physical activity may contribute to weight maintenance or weight loss, in fact, the process is complicated as emphasized in the Consensus Statement on Metabolism from the American Society of Nutrition. Metabolism consists of multiple factors including percent body fat, other issues related to metabolism, and a host of environmental factors.

At any given time, approximately 50%–70% of obese Americans are actively trying to lose weight. Sustained weight loss of as little as 5%–10% is considered clinically significant since it reduces risk factors for a variety of chronic diseases such as CVD and T2DM. Both the Diabetes Prevention Program and the Look AHEAD Trial showed that weight loss of 7% in individuals with obesity resulted in significant improvement in risk factors for both heart disease and diabetes.

Nutrition represents a cornerstone of treatment for overweight and obesity. Dietary treatments for various diseases have been called medical nutrition therapy (MNT). This therapeutic approach has been used in a variety of medical conditions, but there is strong evidence that MNT improves waist circumference, waist-to-hip ratio, fasting blood sugar, low-density lipoprotein cholesterol, high-density lipoprotein cholesterol, and blood pressure.

Typical nutritional interventions for weight loss in individuals with obesity involve sustaining an average daily caloric deficit of 500 kcal. Energy recommendations also include that lower intake should not be less than 1,200 calories/day for male or female adults in order to maintain adequate nutrient intake.

A variety of evidence-based diets have been demonstrated to assist in healthy weight loss. These include the Mediterranean diet, the DASH diet, and the Healthy U.S. Eating Style Pattern. It has been demonstrated that macronutrient composition of a weight loss plan (e.g. low fat versus low carb) does not achieve different results in studies lasting longer than one year.

Weight loss guidelines currently issued by the U.S. Preventive Services Task Force, the American Heart Association, the American College of Cardiology, The Obesity Society, and the Academy of Nutrition and Dietetics all recommend a multidisciplinary team approach to managing patients with obesity. These approaches include physical activity, counseling, MNT, and a structured approach to behavior change utilizing problem solving and goal setting as well as self-monitoring. Most evidence suggests that an effective weight loss program should last at least six months and have a minimum of 24 counseling sessions.

There is a prevalent misconception, particularly amongst physicians, that maintenance of weight loss is virtually impossible. However, in both the Diabetes Prevention Program and the Look AHEAD Trial, individuals who completed the initial 16-week program and then were followed on a monthly basis for the next 3–4 years were able to maintain 90% of the weight that they initially lost. The National Weight Control Registry, which is a registry of over 10,000 individuals who have lost at least 50 pounds and kept it off for at least one year, demonstrated that components of lifestyle measures such as regular attention to monitoring nutritional intake as well as regular physical activity (on average 60 minutes/day) were key to how these individuals were able to maintain initial weight loss.

It has been argued that physical activity alone is not a powerful tool for initial weight loss. While this may be true, abundant evidence supports the concept that regular physical activity is a key component of long-term maintenance of weight loss. Regular physical activity, in combination with energy restriction, has been repeatedly shown to be effective for short-term weight loss. In addition, regular physical activity also plays an important role in the preservation of lean body mass which is a key component for maintaining adequate metabolism to support the maintenance of weight loss. Regular physical activity also conveys a host of health-enhancing benefits in addition to its role in weight loss and weight management.

For all the above reasons, we hope that the current book will prove valuable to all clinicians working in the weight loss area as well as primary care physicians who include weight loss and weight management as an important part of their overall clinical practice. The current book intends to cover a variety of important areas related to modern understandings in the management of obesity. The first 11 chapters of the book explore current understandings of the scope of the problem of obesity and the underlying pathophysiology of the condition. Several chapters also emphasize how various lifestyle modalities such as dietary interventions, exercise, and behavioral management also impact on the effective treatment of obesity. Pharmacologic management and surgery are also emphasized in separate chapters. An individual chapter is focused on managing childhood obesity and a new diagnostic term "adiposity based chronic disease" (ABCD) is also outlined in its own separate chapter.

The next five chapters explore the relationship of obesity to various chronic diseases such as cardiovascular disease (CVD), type 2 diabetes (T2DM), metabolic syndrome (MetS), cancer, and arthritis. The third section contains a separate chapter devoted to an exploration of how different types and locations of adipose tissue contribute to its interaction with chronic diseases. The book closes with chapters on how obesity interacts with public health and future directions in obesity and weight management.

The challenges of writing a book that spans modern knowledge about obesity all the way from basic pathophysiology to its clinical treatment were facilitated by a distinguished group of scientists and clinicians. We challenged all of our collaborating authors to blend state-of-the-art knowledge in basic science with a particular emphasis on clinical applications. Our emphasis is on clinically relevant information which will be of benefit to the practicing physician and other healthcare workers.

We hope and believe that what has emerged is a state-of-the-art body of information about the modern understandings of obesity – both its prevention and treatment. We hope and believe that this book will guide physicians, nurses, nutritionists, exercise physiologists, and other healthcare workers as well as students in these disciplines as they take steps to prevent obesity and/or, if already present, treat it and associated conditions. Our strong emphasis on lifestyle measures fits in with the emerging field of lifestyle medicine which we hope will make this book particularly relevant to healthcare professionals as they understand the power of lifestyle measures and practices in obesity treatment.

The worldwide epidemic of obesity and its comorbidities demands best practices and commitment on the part of healthcare workers. We hope and believe that this book will help clinicians combat this major worldwide epidemic.

James M. Rippe, MD
Boston, Massachusetts

John P. Foreyt, PhD
Houston, Texas

Acknowledgments

Numerous individuals have made significant contributions to all phases of writing, editing, and producing this textbook and deserve our recognition and gratitude.

First, we wish to thank and acknowledge the outstanding work of every chapter author in the book. We hope and believe that the efforts of these distinguished scientists will help bridge the gap between basic science and clinical practice in the prevention and treatment of obesity.

We would also like to acknowledge Dr. Rippe's Managing Editor, Elizabeth Grady. Beth coordinates multiple publications for health care professionals including numerous major textbooks, two academic journals, and numerous books and publications for the general public. Beth has enormous skills, unparalleled work ethic, and phenomenal organizational skills. She manages to coordinate work with multiple publishers and authors, all the while maintaining a sense of calm and good humor.

Dr. Rippe's Executive Assistant, Carol Moreau and Office Assistant, Deb Adamonis coordinate and manage his complex professional and personal life and create the space for the substantial amount of time required to write and edit books.

Our editor at Taylor & Francis Group/CRC Press, Randy Brehm, Senior Editor, who has been an early champion of lifestyle medicine books.

Julia Tanner, Editorial Assistant, in the Life Sciences and Medical Group at CRC Press handled the many details of this book prior to publication.

Marsha Hecht, Project Editor at the Taylor and Francis Group who was responsible for the overall production of this book and Rajamalar Rathnasekar, Project Manager at codeMantra, who handled the day to day production of the book.

Finally, our families continue to support our efforts with unfailing encouragement and love to them and the many others who helped and too numerous to count, we are deeply grateful.

Editors

Dr. Rippe is a cardiologist and graduate of Harvard College and Harvard Medical School with postgraduate training at Massachusetts General Hospital. He is currently the Founder and Director of the Rippe Lifestyle Institute and Professor of Medicine at the University of Massachusetts Medical School.

Over the past 25 years Dr. Rippe has established and run the largest research organization in the world exploring how daily habits and actions impact short and long-term health and quality of life. This organization, Rippe Lifestyle Institute (RLI), has published hundreds of papers that form the scientific basis for the fields of lifestyle medicine and high-performance health. Rippe Lifestyle Institute also conducts numerous studies every year on physical activity, nutrition, and healthy weight management.

Dr. Rippe and the research team at RLI have written over 500 academic publications and written or edited 56 books including 36 books for the medical and health care community and 20 books for the general public. He has published extensively in the areas of cardiovascular medicine, physical activity, nutrition, and weight management.

A lifelong and avid athlete Dr. Rippe maintains his personal fitness with a regular walk, jog, swimming, and weight training program. He holds a black belt in karate and is an avid wind surfer, skier, and tennis player. He lives outside of Boston with his wife, television news anchor Stephanie Hart, and their four children, Hart, Jaelin, Devon, and Jamie.

John P. Foreyt received his PhD in clinical psychology in 1969 from Florida State University. He served on the faculty there until 1974 when he moved to Baylor College of Medicine, Houston, Texas. He is currently Professor at the Baylor College of Medicine's Department of Medicine and Department of Psychiatry. He is also the Director of the DeBakey Heart Center's Behavioral Medicine Research Center.

Dr. Foreyt has served as a member of the National Task Force on the Prevention and Treatment of Obesity, National Institutes of Health; The Committee to Develop Criteria for Evaluating the Outcomes of Approaches to Prevent and Treat Obesity, Food and Nutrition Board, Institute of Medicine, National Academy of Sciences; and The Expert Panel on the Identification, Evaluation, and Treatment of Overweight and Obesity in Adults, National Institutes of Health, NHLBI.

He is a member of the editorial boards of *Obesity Research and Clinical Practice*; *American Journal of Lifestyle Medicine*; *American Journal of Health Behavior*; *Obesity and Weight Management*; *American Journal of Health Promotion*; *Childhood Obesity*; and *Nutrition Today*.

Dr. Foreyt is an Overseas Fellow of the Royal Society of Medicine, a Fellow of the Society of Behavioral Medicine, a Fellow of The Obesity Society, and a Fellow of the Academy of Behavioral Medicine Research. He is a Life Member of the American Psychological Association and an honorary member of the Academy of Nutrition and Dietetics.

Contributors

Katherine R. Arlinghaus, PhD, RD
Division of Epidemiology and
  Community Health, School of
  Public Health
University of Minnesota
Minneapolis, Minnesota

Nina Crowley, PhD, RDN, LD
Metabolic & Bariatric Surgery Program
  Coordinator
Medical University of South Carolina
Charleston, South Carolina

Nikhil V. Dhurandhar, PhD, FTOS
Department of Nutritional Sciences
Texas Tech University
Lubbock, Texas

John P. Foreyt, PhD
Department of Medicine
Baylor College of Medicine
Houston, Texas

Robert F. Kushner, MD
Center for Lifestyle Medicine
Northwestern University Feinberg
  School of Medicine
Chicago, Illinois

Magdalena Pasarica, MD, PhD
College of Medicine
University of Central Florida
Orlando, Florida

James M. Rippe, MD
Rippe Lifestyle Institute
Shrewsbury, Massachusetts
and
University of Massachusetts Medical
  Center
Worcester, Massachusetts

Section I

The Modern Management of Obesity

1 Preventing and Managing Obesity
The Scope of the Problem

James M. Rippe, MD
Rippe Lifestyle Institute
University of Massachusetts Medical School

CONTENTS

1.1 INTRODUCTION

Obesity is a pandemic which represents one of the most significant public health issues for the world in recent history. It is currently estimated that 2.1 billion people in the world are obese [1]. Furthermore, obesity significantly contributes to both worldwide morbidity and mortality [2]. In 2013, obesity was recognized by the American Medical Association as a disease. Furthermore, research supports that obesity increases the risk for many chronic diseases including cardiovascular disease (CVD), cancer, type 2 diabetes (T2DM), metabolic syndrome (MetS), chronic kidney disease, and many musculoskeletal conditions.

The prevalence of obesity in the United States has been increasing for almost 100 years [3]. Since the 1960s, the National Health and Nutrition Examination Survey (NHANES) has taken an active role in tracking obesity in the United States [4,5]. The prevalence of obesity remained fairly constant between 1960 and 1980. However, according to the NHANES data, in each interval from 1976 to 1980 and 1988 to 1994 the prevalence of adult obesity increased by eight percentage points. Recent data suggest that obesity plateaued with no significant increase in prevalence in the United States in the interval between 2003 and 2010, but increased in the intervals from 2005 to 2006 and 2013 to 2014 [6,7]. The current prevalence of obesity is more than double that of 1970 with 42.5% of the population considered obese and 73.6% considered overweight or obese in the United States

DOI: 10.1201/9781003099116-2

1.2   THE BURDEN OF OVERWEIGHT AND OBESITY IN THE UNITED STATES

Childhood obesity represents a relatively new chronic disease epidemic with significant medical and health implications. The prevalence of children with obesity has increased significantly since the 1980s, paralleling the increase in adults with obesity during this period [8]. The prevalence of obesity among 2–19 year olds in the United States is 18.5% and continues to rise across all age groups. Obesity disproportionately affects black, Hispanic, and other minority youths. Comorbid conditions such as T2DM are projected to increase dramatically as generations of children carry obesity into adulthood.

In addition to the enormous health toll attributable to obesity, the obesity epidemic is also driving enormous costs. It is estimated in the United States, for example, that obesity may cost as much as $147 billion each year [9]. Roughly one-half of this total is paid by the government (i.e. taxpayers), and the other half is paid by private insurers. Thus, taxes and employee premiums (paid by all employees, regardless of weight) finance much of the cost of treating obesity and its related conditions.

It is estimated that an individual with obesity costs a health plan 47% more in healthcare expenditures and an individual who is overweight costs the health plan 16% more annually than healthy weight individuals. For all of these reasons, multiple stakeholders including governments, employers, taxpayers, and employees all have significant motivation to slow down rising rates of obesity, if only for its financial impact.

It is clear that obesity is a complicated, multifactorial problem with numerous external and internal influences which impact obese individuals. There is no question that in the United States, and in most of the Western world, we live in an obesogenic environment (it has even been called a "toxic" environment) for weight gain. There are multiple factors that impact weight gain and obesity including family, culture, community, government, and world food policies. There is also clearly an influence from genetics since some individuals are more likely to gain weight than others and some ethnic groups (e.g. black and Hispanic women) are more affected than others [9,10].

The recognition that obesity is an urgent national imperative has been articulated by multiple evidence-based documents. Perhaps the most prominent of these are the Dietary Guidelines for Americans 2020–2025, which characterize obesity as the leading nutritional health problem in our country [11]. The Physical Activity Guidelines for Americans 2018 (PAGA 2018) comes to similar conclusions. The goal of limiting obesity to no more than 15% of the adult population was articulated in the Healthy People 2020 document [12] and again in the 2030 document [13]. In the 2020 document, this was clearly wishful thinking. The United States is moving away from this goal rather than toward it.

For all these reasons, it is no longer a viable option for healthcare professionals to stay on the sidelines, both as individual practitioners and community leaders, when it comes to the urgent problems of both adults and children with obesity. This is the underlying premise behind the current book.

1.3 HEALTH EFFECTS OF OBESITY

- *Role of adipocytes*: It used to be thought that adipocytes were primarily storage sites for excess fat. Research over the last two decades, however, has clarified that adipocytes are, in fact, highly complicated inflammatory, endocrine, and metabolic cells [14–17]. Essentially, adipose tissue thus serves as a complicated endocrine organ and a potent source of inflammatory molecules such as IL-6, Tumor Necrosis Factor alpha (TNFα), and many others [15]. The complex properties of adipocytes appear to underlie the strong relationship between obesity and a variety of chronic medical conditions such as coronary heart disease (CHD), T2DM, and MetS. The complex metabolic and inflammatory properties of adipocytes seem particularly prominent in those located in the abdominal region.
- *Health effects in adults*: The adverse health consequences of obesity are diverse and profound. As already indicated, obesity is strongly associated with T2DM (see Chapter 13), metabolic syndrome (see Chapter 14), CHD (see Chapter 12), and some cancers (see Chapter 15), as well as arthritis (see Chapter 16). This list of adverse health consequences of obesity is by no means exhaustive. A more complete listing is found in Table 1.1.

It has been argued that unless we can control the twin epidemics of obesity and diabetes, the mortality of these two interrelated adverse health conditions could potentially wipe out all of the other gains in the prevention of cardiovascular disease over the past 20 years. According to an article by Ford et al., there were an estimated 149,635 fewer deaths from cardiovascular disease (CVD) occurring between 1980 and 2000 as a result of the decrease in prevalence of major risk factors [18]. An estimated 59,370 additional deaths from diseases, however, occurred because of high rates of obesity and diabetes. These data are depicted graphically in Figure 1.1.

- Health effects in children: While the manifestations of many metabolic diseases occur in middle age or later years, a large body of research now supports that events or conditions that occur in childhood, or perhaps even before birth, can significantly influence the risk of obesity [19,20], T2DM, and CHD. In addition, the risk of a child with obesity increases the risk of becoming an adult with obesity. It has now been estimated that over half of new cases of diabetes in children are T2DM which used to be called "adult onset diabetes," but now is increasingly found in the pediatric population. Furthermore, adolescents with obesity carry a significant increase of severe obesity in adulthood.

1.4 SEARCHING FOR SOLUTIONS

Given the complexity of multiple underlying causes for the obesity epidemic, it is unlikely that a single solution will resolve this problem. For this reason, a number of organizations have proposed frameworks looking at multiple levels of influencers where intervention could help with this issue.

TABLE 1.1
Medical Conditions Associated with Obesity

- *Metabolic Conditions*
  Type 2 diabetes
  Metabolic syndrome
  Glucose intolerance
  Cardiovascular disease
  CHD
  Stroke
  Heart failure
  Deep venous thrombosis
- *CHD Risk Factors*
  Dyslipidemia
  Hypertension
  Inflammation
  Hypercoagulability
- *Pulmonary Disease*
  Obstructive sleep apnea
  Hypoventilation syndrome
  Asthma
  Cancers
  Colorectal
  Esophageal
  Endometrial
  Breast (postmenopausal)
  Kidney
- *Gastrointestinal Diseases*
  Nonalcoholic fatty liver disease
  Gallstones cholecystitis
  Gastroesophageal reflux
- *Other Conditions*
  Gout
  Kidney stones
  Osteoarthritis
  Psychological disorders
  Fertility and pregnancy complications
  Erectile dysfunction

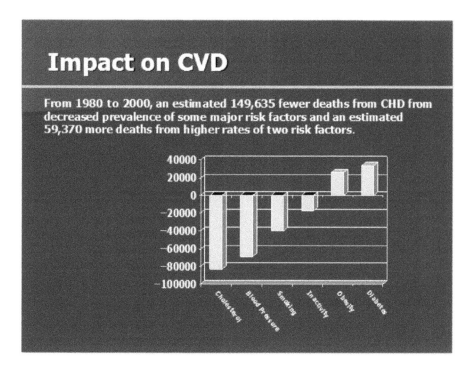

FIGURE 1.1   From 1980 to 2000, an estimated 149,635 fewer deaths occurred from decreased prevalence of some major risk factors and an estimated 59,370 more deaths from higher rates of two risk factors. (From Ford, E.S. et al., *N. Engl. J. Med.*, 256, 2388, July 2007.)

- *Socioeconomic framework*: One framework for approaching obesity and weight management was proposed by the Dietary Guidelines for Americans Advisory Committee 2010 [21,22]. This is depicted in Figure 1.2.

  This framework underscores the concept that energy balance is a complicated issue influenced by multiple and complex factors. This framework can provide a basis for interventions at multiple levels to address the obesity epidemic.

- *Food environment*: It is important to maintain a comprehensive approach to the modern food environment when addressing obesity. In the United States, for example, the average food consumption increased dramatically over the past four decades. As depicted in Figure 1.3, the average daily caloric consumption in the United States increased from 2057 calories in 1970–2674 kcal in 2008.

  This trend has continued to the present time. It has been argued by Swinburne and others that increased caloric consumption in the United States in the past four decades is more than sufficient to explain the U.S. epidemic of obesity [23]. Other investigators have disputed this argument and have pointed to diminished physical activity and other aspects of the environment which have also contributed in a significant way to the obesity

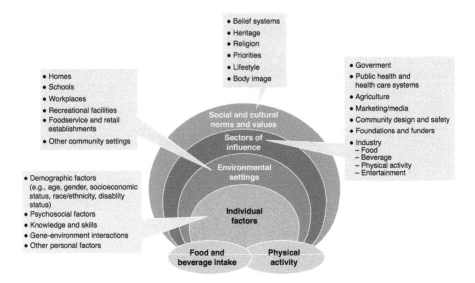

FIGURE 1.2   The socioeconomic framework impacting on energy balance. (Adapted from Dietary Guidelines https://health.gov/sites/default/files/2020-01/DietaryGuidelines2010.pdf. Accessed August 24, 2020.)

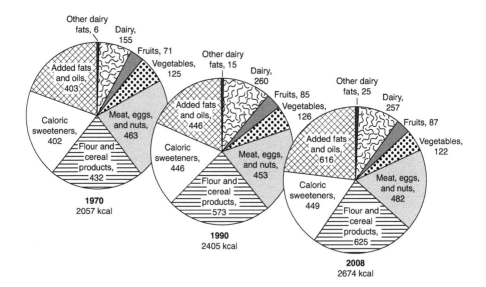

FIGURE 1.3   Average daily per capita calories from the U.S. food availability in 1970, 1990, and 2008, adjusted for spoilage and other waste. From ERS Food Availability. (Per Capita Data System, https://www.ers.usda.gov/data-products/food-availability-per-capita-data-system/.)

epidemic. It also should be noted that recommendations from the Dietary Guidelines for Americans 2015–2020 and 2020–2025 are not being followed by the majority of Americans. In particular, there are substantial shortfalls in fruits, non-fat dairy and vegetables, as well as whole grains.

- *Physical activity*: Unfortunately, the United States population has become increasingly inactive. The Physical Activity Guidelines for Americans 2018 (PAGA 2018) noted that less than 25% of American adults achieve recommended levels of physical activity recommended by the PAGA 2018 and multiple other organizations of 150 minutes of moderate-intensity physical activity per week. According to the PAGA 2018 Scientific Report, only 25% of individuals achieve this level of physical activity [24]. Multiple studies have shown that physically active people are at reduced risk of becoming overweight or obese. In addition, of course, there are multiple other benefits of physical activity (see also Chapter 5).
- *Genetics*: Genetics also plays an important role in the modern obesity epidemic. The "thrifty gene hypothesis" posits that over many millennia human beings survived who had a genetic makeup that allowed them to continue to survive during periods of low food supply [9,10]. In the modern environment, however, this genetic makeup has become maladaptive since it can contribute to individuals storing excess calories as fat in a world where the food supply is abundant in many countries. Multiple lines of evidence including twin studies have also underscored that a significant genetic component exists concerning why some individuals have more problems controlling weight than others. It has been estimated that up to 40% of both children and adults with obesity may be attributed to genetic factors. It should be noted that this leaves a large component of weight gain and obesity to lifestyle habits and practices making it all the more important for individuals who are susceptible to weight gain to maintain particular vigilance of food and exercise choices.

  Exploration of specific areas of genetic contributions to controlling food intake, physical activity, and weight gain are under active investigation. Researchers anticipate that there will be a time when genetics research will yield important answers to help weight control become more individualized and precise.
- *Closing the energy gap*: Blackburn et al. have suggested that healthcare professionals should focus first on individuals with extreme obesity (BMI ≥ 40 kg/m^2) since this is the segment of the obese population that is increasing at rates faster than any other class of obesity in the United States [25]. These investigators also suggest that a useful construct in guiding interventions in these individuals is the "energy gap." They estimate that an energy gap of approximately 400 kcal/day now exists, which was not present in the 1970s. They further argue that closing this excess energy gap should be the highest priority for treating individuals with severe obesity. Blackburn et al. suggest that a lifestyle approach involving improved dietary composition, calorie restriction, and increased physical activity as key components of the lifestyle intervention to close this energy gap.

- *Small step approach:* A report on energy balance and obesity from the American Society of Nutrition has argued that current initiatives designed to combat obesity have not succeeded in reversing the obesity epidemic. This panel presented an alternative strategy of not focusing on weight loss but promoting small changes in physical activity to initially prevent further weight gain [26]. This type of approach is supported by a variety of lines of evidence and appears to hold some promise to combat obesity.

1.5   NEED FOR HEALTHCARE PROFESSIONAL INVOLVEMENT

Given the multiple, negative health consequences of obesity and its high prevalence around the world, it is critically important to healthcare professionals to become actively involved and knowledgeable in multiple aspects of this issue. This is the basic underlying premise for this book. Our goal is to provide modern understandings of obesity as well as specific tools and practical applications for clinicians to use in their daily practices. With this in mind, we will provide general guidance for diagnosing and treating obesity as well as the relationship between weight gain and obesity to a variety of different medical conditions.

One good place to start are guidelines issued in 2013 from the American College of Cardiology (ACC), the American Heart Association (AHA), and The Obesity Society (TOS) [27]. These guidelines recommend a series of steps starting with obtaining the vital signs of obesity including weight, body mass index (BMI), and waist circumference. The guidelines then proceed to recommend comprehensive treatments including nutritional recommendations as well as guidance for physical activity.

Despite the widespread understanding that obesity carries multiple health risks, clinicians have not been appropriately aggressive in counseling individuals to either prevent obesity or help in weight loss for obese individuals. In fact, less than 40% of physicians counsel patients in these areas. This is a wasted opportunity since over 70% of individuals see their primary care physician at least once a year [28].

1.6   SUMMARY/CONCLUSIONS

The prevalence of obesity has continued to rise over the last 40 years throughout the world. In fact, it is now estimated that there are over two billion individuals around the world with obesity, and this is projected to continue to rise for the foreseeable future. Obesity is clearly associated with other metabolic diseases such as CHD, T2DM, MetS, and a number of different cancers. Obesity creates a total body inflammatory condition. For all of these reasons, proper diagnosis and treatment of obesity is a critically important aspect of evidence-based medicine.

1.6.1   Clinical Applications

- Clinicians should obtain vital signs of obesity on all patients including body weight, BMI, and waist circumference.

- A variety of tools are available to help clinicians counsel patients in the area of obesity including recent guidance from the American Heart Association, the American College of Cardiology, and The Obesity Society.
- Obesity is a multifactorial condition that is influenced not only by the individual him/herself and their family, but also by the community, food environment, and many other influences. All of these should be taken into account by clinicians.

REFERENCES

1. Ng M., Fleming T., Robinson M., et al. Global, regional, and national prevalence of overweight and obesity in children and adults during 1980–2013: A systematic analysis for the global burden of disease study 2013. *Lancet (London, England).* 2014;384(9945):766–781.
2. Anonymous. Clinical guidelines on the identification, evaluation, and treatment of overweight and obesity in adults—The evidence report. National Institutes of Health. *Obesity Research.* 1998;6(Suppl 2):51S–209S.
3. Heimburger D., Allison D., Goran M., et al. A festschrift for Roland L. Weinsier: Nutrition scientist, educator, and clinician. *Obesity Research.* 2003;11(10):1246–1262.
4. Flegal K., Carroll M., Kuczmarski R., et al. Overweight and obesity in the United States: Prevalence and trends, 1960–1994. *International Journal of Obesity and Related Metabolic Disorders: Journal of the International Association for the Study of Obesity.* 1998;22(1):39–47.
5. Kuczmarski R., Flegal K., Campbell S., et al. Increasing prevalence of overweight among US adults. The National Health and Nutrition Examination Surveys, 1960 to 1991. *The Journal of the American Medical Association.* 1994;272(3):205–211.
6. Flegal K., Carroll M., Kit B., et al. Prevalence of obesity and trends in the distribution of body mass index among US adults, 1999–2010. *The Journal of the American Medical Association.* 2012;307(5):491–497.
7. Flegal K., Kruszon-Moran D., et al. Trends in obesity among adults in the United States, 2005 to 2014. *The Journal of the American Medical Association.* 2016;315(21):2284–2291.
8. Ogden C., Carroll M., Kit B., et al. Prevalence of childhood and adult obesity in the united states, 2011–2012. *The Journal of the American Medical Association.* 2014;311(8):806–814.
9. Flegal K., Carroll M., Ogden C., et al. Prevalence and trends in obesity among US adults, 1999–2008. *The Journal of the American Medical Association.* 2010;303(3):235–241.
10. Speakman J., Rance K., Johnstone A. Polymorphisms of the FTO gene are associated with variation in energy intake, but not energy expenditure. *Obesity (Silver Spring, Md.).* 2008;16(8):1961–1965.
11. U.S. Department of Agriculture and U.S. Department of Health and Human Services. Dietary Guidelines for Americans, 2020–2025. 9th Edition. December 2020. Available at DietaryGuidelines.gov.
12. US Department of Health and Human Services. Healthy People 2020 objectives. Washington, DC: Department of Health and Human Services, 2010. Available at: http://www.healthypeople.gov/2020/topicsobjectives2020/pdfs/HP2020objectives.pdf.
13. US Department of Health and Human Services. Office of Disease Prevention and Health Promotion. Healthy People 2030. Available at: https://health.gov/healthypeople.
14. Wajchenberg B.L. Subcutaneous and visceral adipose tissue: Their relation to the metabolic syndrome. *Endocrine Reviews* 2000;21:697–738.

15. Hotamisligil G.S., Arner P., Caro J.F., Atkinson R.L., Spiegelman B.M. Increased adipose tissue expression of tumor necrosis factor-alpha in human obesity and insulin resistance. *Journal of Clinical Investigation* 1995;95:2409–2415.
16. Lundgren C.H., Brown S.L., Nordt T.K., Sobel B.E., Fujii S. Elaboration of type-1 plasminogen activator inhibitor from adipocytes: A potential pathogenetic link between obesity and cardiovascular disease. *Circulation* 1996;93:106–110.
17. Yudkin J.S., Stehouwer C.D., Emeis J.J., Coppack S.W. C-reactive protein in healthy subjects: associations with obesity, insulin resistance, and endothelial dysfunction: A potential role for cytokines originating from adipose tissue? *Arteriosclerosis, Thrombosis, and Vascular Biology* 1999;19:972–978.
18. Ford E.S., Ajani U.A., Croft J.B., Critchley J.A., Labarthe D.R., Kottke T.E., Giles W.H., Capewell S. Explaining the decrease in US deaths from coronary disease, 1980–2000. *The New England Journal of Medicine* 2007;256:2388–2398.
19. Biro F.M., Wien M. Childhood obesity and adult morbidities. *The American Journal of Clinical Nutrition.* 2010;91:1499S–1505S.
20. Wardle J., Carnell S., Haworth C., Plomin R. Evidence for a strong genetic influence on childhood adiposity despite the force of the obesogenic environment. *The American Journal of Clinical Nutrition* 2008;87:398–404.
21. Report of the Dietary Guidelines Advisory Committee on the Dietary Guidelines for Americans, US Department of Agriculture, Center for Nutrition Policy and Promotion. Washington, DC. June 2010. https://health.gov/sites/default/files/2020-01/DietaryGuidelines2010.pdf
22. ERS Food Availability (per capita) Data System. http://www.ers.usda.gov/Data/Food Consumption/
23. Swinburne B., Sacks G., Ravussin E. Increased food energy supply is more than sufficient to explain the US epidemic of obesity. *The American Journal of Clinical Nutrition* 2009;90:1453–1456.
24. 2018 Physical Activity Guidelines Advisory Committee. 2018 Physical Activity Guidelines Advisory Committee Scientific Report. Washington, DC: U.S. Department of Health and Human Services, 2018.
25. Blackburn G., Wollner S. Heymsfield S.B. Lifestyle interventions for the treatment of class III obesity: A primary target for nutrition medicine in the obesity epidemic. *The American Journal of Clinical Nutrition* 2010;9:289–292.
26. Hill J.O. Can a small-changes approach help address the obesity epidemic? A report of the joint task force of the American society for nutrition, institute of food technologists, and international food information council. *The American Journal of Clinical Nutrition* 2009;89:477–484.
27. Jensen M., Ryan D., Apovian C., et al. *AHA ACC TOS* guideline for the management of overweight and obesity in adults: a report of the American College of Cardiology/*American Heart Association* Task Force on Practice *Guidelines* and The Obesity Society. Circulation. 2014;129(suppl 2):S102–S138.
28. Rippe, J.M. Lifestyle medicine: The health promoting power daily habits and practices. *American Journal of Lifestyle Medicine.* 2018;13:6, 2018.

2 The Pathophysiology of Obesity

James M. Rippe, MD
Rippe Lifestyle Institute
University of Massachusetts Medical School

CONTENTS

2.1 INTRODUCTION

During the past three decades, there has been a dramatic increase in overweight and obesity around the world. The World Health Organization (WHO) now estimates that there are more than 2.1 billion adults with obesity in the world [1]. The prevalence of obesity was 32.2% among adult men and 35.5% among adult women in the United States in 2007–2008 [2].

Obesity is the most prevalent nutritional problem and plays a significant role in multiple chronic diseases including hypertension, cardiovascular disease (CVD), diabetes mellitus (T2DM), and some forms of cancer. Obesity is associated with moderate increases in all-cause mortality and contributes to morbidity and social disadvantage.

Adipose tissue is one of the largest organs in the body [3,4]. Obesity is typically defined as an excess and abnormal accumulation of adipose tissue. Typically, people classified with obesity are 20%–25% heavier than average for men and women.

Body composition measurements are important for clinical perspective and research in obesity. A variety of reliable methodologies is available to obtain accurate measures of total body fat. These include dual-energy X-ray absorptiometry (DEXA), magnetic resonance imaging (MRI), and computer tomography (CT). It is important to recognize, however, that it is difficult and expensive to measure body fat directly. Consequently, obesity is usually defined in large studies as excess body weight rather than excess fat. For example, in epidemiologic studies, body mass index (BMI) which is calculated as weight in kilograms divided by height and meters

DOI: 10.1201/9781003099116-3

13

squared is used as a surrogate for the amount of body fat. BMI correlates well with the risk of chronic diseases.

In addition to the quantity of excess body fat, its distribution within the body is clinically very important. For example, excess fat in the abdomen (central adiposity) is associated with an increased risk of developing CVD, T2DM, breast cancer, and premature death [5,6]. (See also Chapter 13 on beyond subcutaneous fat.) In this chapter, we will review energy balance as well as exploring metabolic parameters of weight gain and discuss the role of adipokines as well as discussing potential contributions of genetics and environment in the development of obesity.

2.2   ENERGY BALANCE

Obesity is the result of an imbalance between energy intake and expenditure. Energy balance is regulated by a complex physiologic system that requires the integration of multiple peripheral signals and coordination in the brain. Obesity is also a multifactorial disease involving the interaction of both environmental and genetic factors that can contribute to disorders of energy balance. Energy balance is usually tightly regulated. Even in societies where obesity is very prevalent the average weight gain is only about 2.2 pounds per year [7]. This reflects an energy excess of about 20 kcal per day or less than 1% of daily energy expenditure.

Humans have a complicated and sophisticated system for regulating energy balance and fat storage in adipocytes. Changes in energy balance sufficient to alter body fat storage trigger a compensatory change in energy intake and energy expenditure, which eventually returns fat storage to its preset level [8]. Obesity develops when energy intake exceeds energy output leading to an accumulation of adipose tissue.

Energy balance is maintained through control of appetite and metabolism. Appetite regulation is complex and affected by the integration of both peripheral and central signals. In the gastrointestinal tract orexin, ghrelin and decreasing concentration of macronutrients (e.g. glucose, fatty acids, and amino acids) stimulate hunger. Following a meal, gastric and duodenal distention creates a feeling of satiety, and this is aided by the release of gastrointestinal peptides such as ghrelin, cholecystokinin (CCK), glucagon-like peptide-1 (GLP-1), and peptide YY3-36 [9].

Food intake is under both short and long-term control. In the short term, hunger develops in response to decreased circulating levels of glucose, fatty acids, and amino acids. Long-term signals depend on the magnitude of energy stores and include the adipose tissue hormone, leptin.

The discovery of the obese (OB) gene and its products greatly enhanced the understanding of physiologic systems regulating energy balance [10]. The OB gene encodes for the leptin hormone, which is secreted by adipocytes in proportion to the level of body adipose mass [11]. Leptin plays a role in regulating energy intake and energy expenditure including appetite and metabolism. Leptin stimulates pathways that promote anorexia and weight loss through a complex series of signaling mechanisms. Low leptin levels trigger a series of events that lead to increased energy intake, whereas high leptin levels are in response to increased fat deposits resulting in a negative energy balance.

There are three main components of energy expenditure. These include resting metabolic rate (RMR), exercise-induced thermogenesis (physical activity), and food-induced thermogenesis [12,13]. RMR contributes 60%–75% of total energy expenditure and depends on lean body mass, energy intake, physical fitness, and other factors such as age, height, stress, and environmental temperature. Dietary thermogenesis is the energy required to digest and store food and is greatest with protein-rich foods. Physical activity is influenced by behavioral and environmental factors. The adrenergic system also plays a major role in regulating energy expenditure.

2.3   METABOLIC PREDICTORS OF WEIGHT GAIN

As already indicated, obesity develops when there is a mismatch between caloric intake and caloric output. A number of techniques have been developed for measuring energy expenditure. The metabolic chamber is considered the most accurate method. The metabolic chamber is a small room where a subject can live for a 24-hour period, while the metabolic rate is measured during meals, sleep and light activities. Researchers measure the heat release (direct calorimetry) from a person's body to determine how much energy each activity has burned in that person. In indirect calorimetry, researchers measure oxygen consumption, carbon dioxide production, and nitrogen excretion to calculate energy expenditure.

The doubly labeled water technique is another method for determining energy expenditure. This is an indirect measurement based on the elimination of deuterium and oxygen from the urine. This method is useful because it allows researchers to measure total carbon dioxide production for a long period (5–20 days) and requires only periodic sampling of urine. This technique is based on measuring the turnover of hydrogen and oxygen into water and carbon dioxide allowing the calculation of energy expenditure. Measuring energy expenditure has been useful in research. In an early study by Ravassin et al., it was determined that individuals with a low rate of energy expenditure may aggregate along with obesity in families suggesting that energy expenditure may have a familial determinate [14]. A number of studies have demonstrated that insulin sensitivity, low fat oxidation, low sympathetic nerve system activity, low plasma level of leptin, fasting insulin, T3, and fasting serum insulin are significant predictors of weight gain.

2.4   FAT CELLS AND ADIPOKINES

Adipose tissue plays an important role in energy homeostasis as well as various physiologic processes and has complex interactions with the brain and peripheral organs. Adipose tissue has been recognized as a major endocrine organ [15,16]. Two types of adipose tissue exist, WAT and VAT. WAT is the predominant type of adipose tissue. Its deposits are found in subcutaneous regions and around visceral or fat and are stored in the form of triglycerides. This adipose tissue constantly communicates with other tissues by the synthesis and release of secretagogues such as leptin, adiponectin, and visfatin which, along with insulin, play an important role in regulating body fat mass.

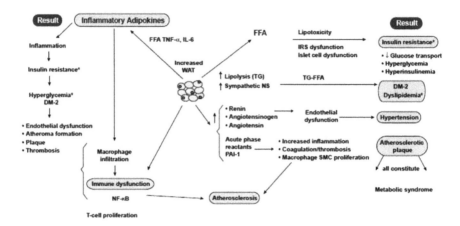

FIGURE 2.1 Role of lipotoxicity and inflammation on obesity. White adipose tissue (WAT) releases pre-fatty acids and adipokines, which are lipotoxic and inflammatory and result in diverse effects, outlined in the left-hand columns. Their correlation to the metabolic syndrome is shown on the right-hand column, whereas all the effects culminate in atherosclerosis at the bottom of the figure. *Perturbed glucose and lipid metabolism. DM-2 = diabetes mellitus-2; FFA = free fatty acids; IL = interleukin; IRS = insulin receptor substrate; NF-xB = nuclear factor kappa beta; NS = nervous system; PAI-l = plasminogen activator inhibitor-1; SMC = smooth muscle cell; TG = triglyceride; TNF = tumor necrosis factor. (Redinger R. The Pathophysiology of Obesity and s. *Gastroenterol Hepatol.* 2007; (NY) Vol 3 (11). Used with permission.)

The pathophysiologic base of obesity is rooted to a large extent in the increased size of fat cells. In the obese state, an increase in WAT brings about several changes characteristic of inflammation that produce inflammatory adipokines such as tumor necrosis factor (TNF), interlukin-6 (IL-6), and interlukin-1 (IL-1) [17,18]. These contribute to vascular dysfunction and, along with free fatty acids, provide a pathophysiologic basis for comorbid conditions associated with obesity such as insulin resistance and T2DM. In addition, C-reactive protein (CRP) is increased in obesity which may induce adhesion and migration of monocytes to WAT endothelium. These conditions eventually may contribute to cardiovascular disease and atherosclerosis [19]. The role of lipotoxicity and inflammation in obesity is depicted in Figure 2.1

2.5 CAUSES OF OBESITY

- *Genetics*: As already indicated, obesity is caused by an imbalance between energy intake and energy expenditure. This process is regulated by complicated physiologic systems. A component of this is the interaction between genetic and environmental factors. An example of this was proposed by James Neel in 1962 with this "thrifty gene hypothesis" [20].

   The genetic component of obesity has been estimated in various studies to be 30%–50%. These studies look at whether or not obesity clusters in family members, twins, and adoptees.

It has been postulated that the genetic component of obesity may be either a single gene (monogenetic obesity) or multiple genes (several genes; polygenic obesity). A variety of genetic approaches looking at segments of DNA have been utilized to begin the process of estimating the genetic component of obesity. Such studies are in their infancy but have considerable potential to contribute to understanding complex diseases including obesity, cancer, T2DM, and CVD.

Monogenic obesity: Several small studies have suggested that there may be a role for monogenic obesity. Single gene defects causing obesity are rare in humans. Several papers have suggested rare mutations in genes including leptin or its receptor [21]. Monogenetic obesity is rare and characterized by extreme phenotype and physiologic perturbation of energy regulation [22,23].

Polygenic obesity: There has been continued progress in identifying multiple genes associated with the most common form of obesity. The theory in polygenic obesity is that an individual's genetic background makes him or her susceptible to an environment that promotes positive energy balance. These studies typically have focused on hundreds of groups of genes related to obesity. These genes are linked to regulatory functions related to fat stores in adipose tissue, energy intake, and energy expenditure. Approximately 500 variants of 130 genes have been associated with obesity [24–26]. Several independent population studies report that the FTO gene (fat mass and obesity-associated gene) might be responsible for up to 22% of common obesity in the general population [27]. It is also possible that a particular genotype may be expressed only under certain adverse environmental conditions such as high-fat diets and sedentary lifestyles in the United States as well as other western countries.

- *Environment*: While, as already indicated, genetic contributions to obesity have been given recent considerable attention, the dramatic increase in the prevalence of obesity over the last three decades is most likely due to environmental changes and effects [28]. Thus, individuals who are genetically susceptible are at risk for developing obesity in an environment that promotes high energy intake of food and low energy expenditure (e.g. physical inactivity). Rapid increase in the mean population of obesity can only be caused by such environmental influences that disturb the basic homeostatic mechanisms already described in this chapter.

Caloric density: In the last three decades, there has been a significant increase in consumption of energy-dense food and soft drinks that are high in fat and/or sugar [29–31]. From the early 1970s to 2010, the average caloric consumption in the United States increased by over 500 calories per day. Total calorie consumption has increased around the world and has been found to be related to obesity. Of particular concern is the association between fast-food consumption and obesity [32]. The USDA reported that the consumption of fast-food meals tripled between 1977 and 1995. The food energy intake from these meals quadrupled during this time period [33].

Physical inactivity: Sedentary lifestyle plays a significant role in obesity [34,35]. According to the Physical Activity Guidelines for Americans 2018 Scientific Report, 75% of adults do not engage in the recommended level of activity and 25%–30% of U.S. adults are not active at all [36]. Similar trends in declining physical activity have been observed worldwide. There are multiple lines of evidence to suggest that physically active people are at reduced risk for weight gain, overweight, and obesity. Promoting regular physical activity and promoting an environment that support this behavior has great potential to reduce the prevalence of obesity as well as other chronic diseases.

2.6   SUMMARY/CONCLUSIONS

The pathophysiology of obesity is based on a mismatch between energy intake and energy expenditure. There are multiple, intricately balanced physiologic processes that interact to maintain a stable weight. However, when these mechanisms are exposed to an environment that promotes increased energy intake and decreased physical activity, the resultant effects are weight gain and, ultimately, obesity. There is also a genetic component of obesity estimated at 30%–50%. However, this genetic component does not explain the dramatic increase in obesity in the United States and worldwide over the past 40 years. Individuals who have a genetic susceptibility to weight gain and obesity should be particularly mindful of lifestyle habits and practices such as paying attention to nutrient-dense, lower-calorie foods and increased physical activity.

PRACTICAL APPLICATIONS

- Energy balance is tightly controlled in human beings.
- If there are perturbations in the energy balance system such as increased consumption of energy-dense foods and lack of physical activity, weight gain and obesity may result.
- There is a genetic component of weight gain and obesity which has been estimated at 30%–50% of the cause of these conditions. This mandates that people who are genetically predisposed to weight gain and obesity should be particularly vigilant about participating in regular physical activity and consuming nutritious foods which are not overly energy dense.

REFERENCES

1. Ng M., Fleming T., Robinson M. Global, regional, and national prevalence of overweight and obesity in children and adults during 1980–2013: A systematic analysis for the Global Burden of Disease Study 2013. *The Lancet*. 2014;384:766–81.
2. Flegal K., Carroll M., Ogden C., et al. Prevalence and trends in obesity among US adults, 1999–2008. *JAMA*. 2010;303(3):235–41.
3. Cohen D., Finch B., Bower A., et al. Collective efficacy and Obesity: The potential influence of social factors on health. *Soc. Sci. Med.* 2006;62(3):769–78.

4. Gray L., Hart C., Smith G., et al. What is the predictive value of established risk factors for total and cardiovascular disease mortality when measured before middle age? Pooled analysis of two prospective cohort studies from Scotland. *Eur. J. Cardiovasc. Prev. Rehabil.* 2010;17(1):106–12.

5. Vague J. The degree of masculine differentiation of obesities: A factor determining predisposition to diabetes, atherosclerosis, gout, and uric calculous disease. *Am. J. Clin. Nutr.* 1956;4:20–34.

6. Despres J.-P., Allard C., Tremblay A., et al. Evidence for a regional component of body fatness in the association with serum lipids in men and women. *Metabolism.* 1985;34:967–73.

7. Schwartz M., Woods S., Seeley R. Is the energy homeostasis system inherently biased toward weight gain? *Diabetes* 2003;52:232–8.

8. Kennedy G. The role of depot fat in the hypothalamic control of food intake in the rat. *Proc. R Soc. Lond. (Biol).* 1953;140:579–92.

9. Kumar P., Clarke M.L. *Clinical Medicine*, 5th Edition. Saunders, Ltd., Nottingham, 2002.

10. Zhang Y., Proenca R., Maffel M., et al. Positional cloning of the mouse obese gene and its human homologue. *Nature.* 1994;372:425–32.

11. Green E., Maffei M., Braden V., et al. The human obese (OB) gene: RNA expression pattern and mapping on the physical, cytogenetic, and genetic maps of chromosome 7. *Genome Res.* 1995;5(1):5–12.

12. Olefsky J. Obesity. In: Isselbacher K., Braunwald E., Wilson J.D. (eds.) et al. *Harrison's Principles of Internal Medicine*, 13th edition. New York: McGraw-Hill; 1994:446–52.

13. Zurlo F., Larson K., Bogardus C., Ravussin E. Skeletal muscle metabolism is a major determinant of resting energy expenditure. *J. Clin. Invest.* 1990;86:1423–27.

14. Ravussin E., Lillioja S., Knowler W., et al. Reduced rate of energy expenditure as a risk factor for body-weight gain. *N. Engl. J. Med.* 1988;318:467–72.

15. Butte N., Gai G., Cole S., et al. Metabolic and behavioral predictors of weight gain in Hispanic children: The viva la familia study. *Am. J. Clin. Nutr.* 2007;85:1478–85.

16. Kershaw E., Flier J. Adipose tissue as an endocrine organ. *J. Clin. Endocrinol. Metab.* 2004;89(6):2548–56.

17. Weisberg S., McCann D., Desai M., et al. Obesity is associated with macrophage accumulation in adipose tissue. *J. Clin. Invest.* 2003;112:1796–808.

18. Xu H., Barnes G., Yang Q., et al. Chronic inflammation in fat plays a crucial role in the development of obesity-related insulin resistance. *J. Clin. Invest.* 2003;112:1821–30.

19. Shirai K. Obesity as the core of the metabolic syndrome and the management of coronary heart disease. *Curr. Med. Res. Opin.* 2004;20:295–304.

20. Neel J. Diabetes mellitus: A "thrifty" genotype rendered detrimental by progress? *Am. J. Hum. Genet.* 1962;14:353–62.

21. Montague C., Farooqi I., Whitehead J., et al. Congenital leptin deficiency is associated with severe early-onset obesity in humans. *Nature* 1997;387:903–8.

22. Farooqi I., O'Rahilly S. Monogenic obesity in Humans. *Ann. Rev. Med.* 2005;56:443–58.

23. Hunter D.J. Gene-environment interactions in human diseases. *Nat. Rev. Genet.* 2005;6:287–98.

24. Rankinen T., Zuberi A., Chagnon Y., et al. The human obesity gene map: The 2005 update. *Obesity (Silver Spring)* 2006;14:529–644.

25. Bell C., Walley A., Froguel P. The genetics of human obesity. *Nat. Rev. Genet.* 2005;6: 221–23.

26. Mutch D., Clement K. Unraveling the genetics of human obesity. *PLoS Genet.* 2006;2(12)1956–62.

27. Loos R. Recent progress in the genetics of common obesity. *Br. J. Clin. Pharmacol.* 2009;68:811–29.

28. Ravussin E., Valenci M., Esparza J. et al. Effects of a traditional lifestyle on obesity in pima Indians. *Diabetes Care* 1994;17:1067–974.
29. Flegal K., Carroll M., Ogden C., et al. Prevalence and trends in obesity among US adults, 1999–2000. *JAMA* 2002;288(14):1723–7.
30. Caballero B. The global epidemic of obesity: An overview. *Epidemiol. Rev.* 2007;29:1–5.
31. Mozaffarian D., Hao T., Rimm E., et al. Changes in diet and lifestyle and long-term weight gain in women and men. *New England J. Med.* 2011;364(25):2392–404.
32. Rosenheck R. Fast food consumption and increased caloric intake: A systematic review of a trajectory towards weight gain and obesity risk. *Obes. Rev.* 2008;9(6):535–47.
33. Lin B., Guthrie J., Frazao E. Nutrient contribution of food away from home. In Frazão E. Agriculture Information Bulletin No. 750: America's Eating Habits: Changes and Consequences. Washington, DC: US Department of Agriculture, Economic Research Service. 1999; 213–239.
34. Hu F. Sedentary lifestyle and risk of obesity in type 2 Diabetes. *Lipids* 2003;38(2):103–8.
35. Jacobs R.D. Fast food and sedentary Lifestyle: A combination that leads to obesity. *AJCN* 2006;83(2):189–90.
36. Physical Activity Guidelines Advisory Committee. 2018 Physical Activity Guidelines Advisory Committee Scientific Report. Washington, DC: U.S. Department of Health and Human Services, 2018.

3 The Epidemiology of Adult Obesity

James M. Rippe, MD
Rippe Lifestyle Institute
University of Massachusetts Medical School

CONTENTS

3.1   INTRODUCTION

Obesity is a worldwide pandemic representing enormous public health consequences. It is now estimated that there are 2.1 billion individuals with obesity in the world [1]. Obesity contributes significantly to morbidity and mortality because of its association with multiple chronic diseases.

Obesity increases the risk of multiple chronic disease including cardiovascular disease (CVD), type 2 diabetes (T2DM), cancer, chronic kidney disease, and many musculoskeletal conditions [2]. It has been estimated that over 300,000 deaths in the United States each year are associated with obesity and 2.8 million excess deaths worldwide are attributed to this disease [3,4]. Unfortunately, the rates across the globe continue to increase.

Obesity is a condition characterized by the accumulation of excess adipose tissue. Determining body fat composition is difficult and costly [5]. While there are technologies available to do this such as dual-energy x-ray absorptiometry (DEXA) and bioelectric impedance as well as computer tomography (CT), magnetic resonance imaging (MRI), and ultrasound (UT), as a practical matter these technologies are largely restricted to research organizations and are not used in large-scale epidemiologic studies. Anthropomorphic measurements such as body mass index (BMI), waist circumference (WC), and waist to hip ratio (WHR) are typically utilized in large-scale epidemiologic studies. While each of these anthropomorphic measurements has certain limitations, they provide a good snapshot with regard to overweight and obesity and are reasonably well correlated with both body fat and risk of comorbid conditions.

DOI: 10.1201/9781003099116-4

3.2 PREVALENCE OF OBESITY

BMI is typically used in epidemiologic studies of overweight and obesity because of its affordability and simplicity. BMI allows for standardized tracking and comparison of overweight and obesity within populations.

- *U.S. obesity trends*: The prevalence of obesity has been increasing in the United States for almost 100 years [6]. Since the 1960s, the National Health and Nutrition Examination Survey (NHANES) has taken an active role in tracking the prevalence of obesity in the United States. According to NHANES data, the prevalence of obesity was fairly constant between 1960 and 1980. Between 1980 and 1994, the prevalence of obesity increased by eight percentage points. Recent data have suggested that obesity trends plateaued in the interval between 2003 and 2010, but increased again in the interval between 2006 and 2014 [7]. The current prevalence of obesity, according to NHANES data, is 42.5%, while 73.6% of the population is either overweight or individuals with obesity [8,9]. Every age, ethnicity, and gender group has experienced a significant increase in obesity with all of these segments exceeding 30%.

  More men than women were considered overweight or individuals with obesity (73.9% versus 63.7%). The prevalence of obesity in men remained constant from 2009 to 2014 (35.5% versus 35.2%), but increased for women (36.3%–45%) [8,9]. Obesity prevalence increased significantly for both males and females in all age groups. There are significant variations in the demographic distribution of obesity. The states in the Southeastern and Midwestern United States have higher rates of obesity, although it should be noted that the prevalence of obesity in every state has increased in the past 30 years. In addition, the prevalence of obesity tracks with socioeconomic status (SES). When comparing women of low socioeconomic status to women of higher SES, the prevalence of obesity is 50% higher in women of low SES.
- *Global obesity trends*: Obesity has reached pandemic levels. This is no longer a crisis just for developed countries, but increasingly it is seen also in developing countries. Worldwide the prevalence of obesity among adults has increased by 27.5% from 1980 to 2013 [10–12]. In 1980, 28.8% of men and 29.8% of women were overweight or obese, but by 2013 these numbers had increased to 36.9% and 38.0%, respectively. Evaluation of women in 37 developing countries suggests that lower SES women have had a faster increase in overweight and obesity than have higher SES women [13].
- *Potential causes of obesity*: As discussed in detail in Chapter 2, obesity results from an imbalance between energy intake and expenditure. While this may seem straightforward, it is actually quite complex and relates to metabolic, genetic, environmental, behavioral, cultural, and socioeconomic factors. The leading components of energy imbalance relate to overconsumption of calories and inactivity. Other risk factors may also contribute to this imbalance.

- *Energy imbalance*: When energy intake exceeds energy expenditure, the excess is stored as fat, leading to increased adiposity. Simply reducing energy intake may not be an adequate solution to overweight or obesity since metabolism can slow during energy restriction [14,15]. It should also be noted that energy density for eating occasions has also increased over the past 30 years. Energy expenditure occurs from metabolism, thermoregulation, and daily physical activity. These factors are discussed in more detail in Chapter 2.

- *Genetics and epigenetics*: There is increasing evidence that there is a genetic component to obesity susceptibility [16]. Most research studies have suggested that there is a 30–50% component of genetics with regard to obesity. (See also Chapter 2.)

- *Infections*: There are emerging data that there may be a role for infections in the development of obesity. In some models, up to ten microorganisms have been identified that may relate to obesity [17]. The most prevalent one appears to be adenovirus-36 (Ad-36). The exact mechanism for why Ad-36 is associated with obesity is not well understood. Infections can affect metabolism and impact inflammation, which is a factor associated with obesity. In one meta-analysis, the relationship in humans exposed to Ad-36 add a twofold increase risk of being obese.

- *Smoking*: Smokers have consistently been shown to weigh less than non-smokers. Nicotine is an appetite suppressant and also alters thermogenic responses [18,19]. Of course, cigarette smoking, in and of itself, is a very significant health risk. Current smoking prevalence in the United States has declined from 20.9% in 2005 to 15.1% in 2015, while the prevalence of obesity has increased significantly. Thus, the decreasing prevalence of smoking may be associated with the rising prevalence of overweight and obesity [20]. This is not an argument to smoke cigarettes since this habit yields multiple, serious health risks. However, the two trends seem to have gone in opposite directions.

- *Sleep*: There is some evidence from both human and animal studies that there is an inverse relationship between sleep and obesity. This may be caused by endocrine responses associated with lack of sleep. Sleep deprivation is a risk factor for obesity and should be considered as a component of the overall approach to curbing the obesity epidemic [21,22].

- *Gut microbiota*: Gut microbiota have been shown to play an increasingly prominent role in health including involvement of energy harvesting, storage, metabolic function, and hormonal signaling [23]. Changes in microbiota may lead to an increased capacity for harvesting energy from food. The exact mechanism for how this may lead to obesity is not clearly understood and is an area of active research.

- *Other factors*: Multiple other factors may be involved in the obesity pandemic including endocrine disrupters, pharmaceutical agents, and ambient temperature control. All of these potential factors are subjects of ongoing research.

3.3   HEALTH CONSEQUENCES OF OBESITY

Obesity is associated as a significant risk factor for developing numerous comorbidities. It is also associated with increased overall mortality. Among those conditions that obesity is associated with are an increased risk of CVD, T2DM, numerous cancers, metabolic syndrome (MetS), asthma, chronic back pain, sleep apnea, gout, osteoarthritis, pulmonary embolism, breathing problems, gallbladder disease, pregnancy complications, menstrual irregularities, stress, incontinence, and psychological disorders [24–30]. These comorbidities are handled in various chapters throughout this book. It should also be noted that even small amounts of weight gain as little as 10–12 pounds during adulthood are also associated with increased risk of multiple chronic diseases including CVD and T2DM.

3.4   ECONOMIC COST OF OBESITY IN THE UNITED STATES

Worldwide, the total economic impact of obesity is estimated to be $2 trillion or 2.8% of the gross domestic product [31]. In the United States, obesity is associated with an increased risk of a variety of comorbid conditions such as hypertension, T2DM, and CVD. In addition to these direct costs, obesity is also associated with indirect costs such as presenteeism, absenteeism, disability, and workman's compensation claims [32,33].

- *Direct Costs*: Direct costs of obesity are usually defined as expenses (both out of pocket and insurance coverage) related to services provided by a healthcare provider in a variety of settings. Since obesity is associated with a variety of other conditions such as CVD, hypertension, and T2DM, the treatment of these conditions is factored into the degree to which obesity is associated with them. Utilizing this methodology, a number of studies have suggested obesity is responsible for a large proportion of the cost to the medical system and society. Compared with normal weight individuals, severely obese individuals have 1.5–3.9 times higher direct medical costs. Multiple different studies have attempted to estimate the direct cost of obesity.
- *Indirect costs*: Indirect costs include absenteeism, disability, and worker's compensation claims as well as premature mortality. It has been estimated that the indirect costs of obesity are higher than direct costs and account for 54%–59% of the estimated total costs of obesity. These indirect costs are largely the result of loss of productivity.
  - *Presenteeism and absenteeism*: Presenteeism is defined as time and productivity lost to workers who are at work but are unable to perform at full capacity as a result of obesity-related health problems. In contrast, absenteeism refers to the loss of productivity associated with missed workdays or sick days. A number of studies have shown that obese individuals have a significantly higher probability of missing work compared to workers who are normal weight [34]. In addition, a number

of studies have shown that obese individuals experience more work limitations with regard to time needed to complete tasks and ability to perform job demands. In one study of firefighters, individuals with obesity missed 2.7–5 times the number of workdays (depending on obesity class) compared to normal weight firefighters [35]. Several estimates have been made of incremental costs associated with obesity in both men and women. In men, it has been estimated that between $1,960 and $5,193 extra per year are spent per male worker and between $1,736 and $5,393 extra are spent for female workers compared to normal weight individuals.

- *Disability and premature mortality*: Disability costs result both from short and long-term disability benefits, insurance policies, and government programs. Premature mortality refers to a lower projected life expectancy experienced by obese workers. A number of reviews have shown that obesity is a significant predictor of disability. Other studies have shown that there is a significant relationship between BMI and the number of claims submitted. Total estimated medical and indemnity claims for obese workers have been estimated from one study as $94,125 and $117,107 per 100 full-time equivalent (FTE) workers [36]. At the same time, claim costs for normal weight workers were only $7,503 and $5,396 per 100 FTEs

3.5 SUMMARY/CONCLUSIONS

The prevalence of obesity is very high and represents a global pandemic. Both the economic and health consequences of the continued rise of the obesity epidemic are highly significant. For every reason, a global effort is needed to combat the exceedingly high and growing epidemic of obesity around the world.

CLINICAL APPLICATIONS

- Obesity is associated with multiple chronic comorbidities including cardiovascular disease, type 2 diabetes, some cancers, osteoarthritis, and many others.
- Individuals with obesity should be evaluated not only for their level of obesity, but also the potential for any comorbid conditions.
- Lifestyle measures such as increased physical activity and decreased caloric consumption or decrease in consumption of energy-dense foods should be employed in concert with each other to lower the risk of obesity or assist in healthy weight loss.

REFERENCES

1. Ng M., Fleming T., Robinson, M., et al. Global, regional, and national prevalence of overweight and obesity in children and adults during 1980–2013: A systematic analysis for the global burden of disease study 2013. *Lancet*. 2014; 384:766–781.

2. NHLBI Obesity Education Initiative Expert Panel on the Identification, Evaluation, and Treatment of Overweight and Obesity in Adults. Clinical guidelines on the identification, evaluation, and treatment of overweight and obesity in adults: The evidence report. National Institutes of Health. *Obesity Research*. 1998; 6(Suppl 2):51S–209S.
3. Allison D., Fontaine B., Manson J. Annual deaths attributable to obesity in the United States. *JAMA*. 1999; 282(16):1530–1538.
4. Flegal K., Graubard B., Williamson D., et al. Excess deaths associated with underweight, overweight, and obesity. *JAMA*. 2005; 293(15):1861–1867.
5. Day S., Jitnarin N., Vidoni M. Epidemiology of adult obesity. In Rippe J. (eds.) *Lifestyle Medicine*, 3rd edition. CRC Press, Boca Raton, FL, 2019.
6. Heimburger D., Allison D., Goran M., et al. A festschrift for Roland L. Weinsier: Nutrition scientist, educator, and clinician. *Obesity Research*. 2002; 11 (10):1246–1262.
7. Flegal K., Carroll M., Kit B., Prevalence of obesity and trends in the distribution of body mass index among US adults, 1999–2010. *JAMA*. 2012; 307(5):491–497.
8. CDC: National Center for Health Statistics. Prevalence of Overweight, Obesity, and Severe Obesity Among Children and Adolescents Aged 2–19 Years: United States, 1963–1965 Through 2015–2016 by Fryar CD, Carroll MD, Ogden CL. Division of Health and Nutrition Examination Surveys. https://www.cdc.gov/nchs/data/hestat/obesity_child_15_16/obesity_child_15_16.pdf. Accessed January 2021.
9. Flegal K., Carroll M., Kit B., et al. Prevalence of obesity and trends in the distribution of body mass index among us adults, 1999–2010. *JAMA*. 2012; 307:491–497.
10. Finucane M., Stevens G., Cowan M. National, Regional, and Global trends in body-mass index since 1980: Systematic analysis of health examination surveys and epidemiological studies with 960 country-years and 9.1 million participants. *Lancet*. 2011; 377(9765):557–567.
11. Swinburn B., Sacks G., Hall K., et al. The global obesity pandemic: Shaped by global drivers and local environments. *Lancet*. 2011; 378(9793)804–814.
12. International Association for the Study of Obesity. Global prevalence of adult obesity. In International Association for the Study of Obesity. https://www.omicsonline.org/societies/the-international-association-for-the-study-of-obesity/. Accessed 24 August 2020.
13. Jones-Smith J., Gordon-Larsen P., Siddiqi A., et al. Cross-national comparisons of time trends in overweight inequality by socioeconomic status among women using repeated cross-sectional surveys from 37 developing countries, 1989–2007. *American Journal of Epidemiology*. 2011; 173(6):667–675.
14. Hall K., Sacks G., Chandramohan D., et al. Quantification of the effect of energy imbalance on bodyweight. *Lancet*. 2011; 378(9793):826–837.
15. Hall K., Chow C. Estimating the quantitative relation between food energy intake and changes in body weight. *American Journal of Clinical Nutrition*. 2010; 91(3):816; Author Reply 817.
16. Rankinen T., Zuberi A., Chagnon Y., et al. The human obesity gene map: The 2005 update. *Obesity*. 2006; 14(4):529–644.
17. McAllister E., Dhurandhar N., Keith S., et al. Ten putative contributors to the obesity epidemic. *Critical Reviews in Food Science and Nutrition*. 2009; 49(10):868–913.
18. Filozof C., Fernandez Pinilla M., Fernandez-Cruz A. Smoking cessation and weight gain. *Obesity Reviews*. 2004; 5(2):95–103.
19. Tian J., Venn A., Otahal P., et al. The association between quitting smoking and weight gain: A systemic review and meta-analysis of prospective cohort studies. *Obesity Reviews*. 2015; 16(10):883–901.
20. Chiolero A., Faeh D., Paccaud F., et al. Consequences of smoking for body weight, body fat distribution, and insulin resistance. *The American Journal of Clinical Nutrition*. 2008; 87(4):801–809.

21. Patel S., Malhotra A., White D., et al. Association between reduced sleep and weight gain in women. *American Journal of Epidemiology.* 2006; 164(10):947–954.
22. Patel S., Hu F. Short sleep duration and weight gain: A systematic review. *Obesity.* 2008; 16(3):643–653.
23. Clemente J., Ursell L., Parfrey L., et al. The impact of the gut microbiota on human health: An integrative view. *Cell.* 2012; 148(6):1258–1270.
24. Reis J., Macera C., Araneta M., et al. Comparison of overall obesity and body fat distribution in predicting risk of mortality. *Obesity.* 2009; 17(6):1232–1239.
25. D'Agostino R., Hamman R., Karter A., et al. Cardiovascular disease risk factors predict the development of type 2 diabetes: The insulin resistance atherosclerosis study. *Diabetes Care.* 2004; 27(9):2234–2240.
26. Katzmarzyk P., Janssen I., Ardern C. Physical inactivity, excess adiposity and premature mortality. *Obesity Reviews.* 2003; 4(4):257–290.
27. Kenchaiah S., Gaziano J., Vasan R. Impact of obesity on the risk of heart failure and survival after the onset of heart failure. *The Medical Clinics of North America.* 2004; 88(5):1273–1294.
28. Guh D., Zhang W., Bansback N., et al. The incidence of co-morbidities related to obesity and overweight: A systematic review and meta-analysis. *BMC Public Health.* 2009; 9:88.
29. Wang Y., McPherson K., Marsh T., et al. Health and economic burden of the projected obesity trends in the USA and the UK. *Lancet.* 2011; 378(9793):815–825.
30. Renehan A., Tyson M., Egger M., et al. Body-mass index and incidence of cancer: A systematic review and meta-analysis of prospective observational studies. *Lancet.* 2008; 371(9612): 569–578.
31. Tremmel M., Gerdtham U., Nilsson P., et al. Economic burden of obesity: A systematic literature review. *International Journal of Environmental Research and Public Health.* 2007: 14 (4):435.
32. Dee A., Kearns K., O'Neill C., et al. The direct and indirect costs of both overweight and obesity: A systematic review. *BMC Research Notes.* 2014; 7:242.
33. Grieve E., Fenwick E., Yang H., et al. The disproportionate economic burden associated with severe and complicated obesity: A systematic review. *Obesity Reviews.* 2013; 14(11):883–894.
34. Trogdon J., Finkelstein E., Hylands T., et al. Indirect costs of obesity: A review of the current literature. *Obesity Reviews.* 2008; 9(5):489–500.
35. Poston W., Jitnarin N., Haddock C., et al. Obesity and injury-related absenteeism in a population-based firefighter cohort. *Obesity.* 2011; 19(10):2076–812011.
36. Ostbye T., Dement J., Krause K. Obesity and workers' compensation: Results from the duke health and safety surveillance system. *Archives of Internal Medicine.* 2007; 167(8):766–773.

4 Identification, Evaluation, and Treatment of Overweight and Obesity

James M. Rippe, MD
Rippe Lifestyle Institute
University of Massachusetts Medical School

CONTENTS

4.1 INTRODUCTION

As already indicated, both overweight and obesity are recognized as serious risk factors for overall mortality and multiple metabolic diseases including cardiovascular disease (CVD), diabetes (T2DM), cancer, metabolic syndrome, and many other diseases. For this reason, it is important to evaluate and treat overweight and obesity and other risk factors to reduce the risk of developing comorbid conditions [1,2]. This chapter will focus on the identification and evaluation of patients who are overweight and obese and provide some suggestions for the selection of treatment [3–5]. Both clinical and laboratory information are needed for this evaluation. These practices should be done in the context of a warm, humane, and supportive clinical primary care setting.

4.2 IDENTIFICATION OF OBESITY

At its most fundamental level, obesity refers to an increase in body fat. Unfortunately, measurement of body fat is not easily done in clinical practice. Furthermore, the interpretation of body fatness depends on a variety of factors such as age, gender, ethnic group, nutrition, and level of physical activity.

The importance of distribution of fat is also important. Centrally located fat (i.e. in the abdominal area) has been demonstrated to carry more adverse health

DOI: 10.1201/9781003099116-5

consequences than in the hips or thighs [6]. Central adiposity is a key element in metabolic syndrome and, in turn, cardiovascular disease. Central adiposity is a key component of multiple risk factors for a variety of metabolic diseases including elevated blood pressure, elevated plasma glucose, elevated triglycerides, and low levels of high-density lipoprotein (HDL) cholesterol.

4.3   EVALUATION OF THE OBESE/OVERWEIGHT PATIENT

- *Clinical history*: The clinical history of a patient who is overweight provides basic information which is relevant to assessing the patient's risk for obesity and its metabolic consequences. This includes understanding events that led to the development of overweight or obesity, what the patient has done in the past to deal with the problem, and how successful or unsuccessful he/she has been in these efforts.

   Family history is also important, both because of the attitudes about obesity and the possibility of finding unusual or rare genetic causes. Information concerning the timing and amount of weight gain (>10 kg or >22 lbs) since the age of 18 and the rate of weight gain is important because it relates to the risk of developing complications from obesity. The amount of physical activity is also important since physical inactivity, in addition to contributing to weight gain also increases the risk of CVD. Information about comorbid conditions such as T2DM, hypertension, CVD, sleep apnea, and gallbladder disease also should be obtained.

   A number of drugs can also cause significant weight gain (Table 4.1).

   Further information concerning mental health problems, depression, T2DM, and use of steroids for asthma are also important to obtain. Other potential causes of obesity such as altered menstrual symptoms in women (suggesting polycystic ovary syndrome) or purple-ish abdominal striae (suggesting Cushing's disease).

   Finally, it is important to determine whether or not the patient/client is "ready" to put in the effort to lose weight which will allow the clinician to determine whether the patient is ready at the current time to proceed with treatment.
- *Physical examination*:
  - *Step 1: Measure body mass index*: The clinician or office staff should measure vital signs related to obesity, including height and weight, in order to calculate body mass index (BMI), waist circumference, blood pressure, and any other information related to the patient's complaint. Accurate measurement of height can be obtained using a wall-mounted stadiometer and weight should utilize a regularly calibrated scale in order to calculate BMI. Table 4.2 lists BMI in both height in inches and in centimeters and weight in kilograms or pounds. While BMI does not specifically measure fat, it correlates well with body fat and, more importantly, with health risks. Measurement of BMI provides an excellent starting point for counseling the overweight or obese individual.

TABLE 4.1
Drugs that Produce Weight Gain and Alternatives

Category	Drugs that Cause Weight Gain	Possible Alternatives
Neuroleptics	Thioridazine, olanzapine, quetiapine, risperidone, clozapine	Molindone, haloperidol, ziprasidone
Anti-depressants	Amitriptyline, nortriptyline	Protriptyline
Tricyclics	Imipramine	Bupropion, nefazadone
Monoamine oxidase inhibitors	Mirtazapine	Fluoxetine, sertraline
Selective serotonin reuptake inhibitors	Paroxetine	
Anti-convulsants	Valproate, carbamazepine, gabapentin	Topiramate, lamotrigine, zonisamide
Anti-diabetic drugs	Insulin	Acarbose, miglitol, sibutramine
	Sulfonylureas	Metformin, orlistat
	Thiazolidinediones	
Anti-serotonin	Pizotifen	
Antihistamines	Cyproheptidine	Inhalers, decongestants
β-Adrenergic blockers	Propranolol	Angiotensin-converting enzyme
α-Adrenergic blockers	Terazosin	inhibitors, calcium channel blockers
Steroid hormones	Contraceptives	Barrier methods
	Glucocorticoids	Non-steroidal anti-inflammatory agents
	Progestational steroids	

Bray G: Identification, evaluation and treatment of obesity. In Rippe JM, Angelopoulos TJ. *Obesity Prevention and Treatment*, CRC Press (Boca Raton), 2012. Reprinted from Obesity Prevention and Treatment by Rippe JM and Angelopoulos, TJ. CRC Press (Boca Raton), 2012. Used with permission of the Editor Dr. James M. Rippe, MD.

- *Step 2: Measure waist circumference*: Waist circumference is the most practical approach to estimating visceral fat [7,8] Waist circumference is measured with a flexible tape placed horizontally at the level of the superior iliac crest [9]. The current classification of obesity based on BMI and waist circumference as recommended by the National Heart, Lung and Blood Institute (NHLBI) and the World Health Organization (WHO) are shown in Table 4.3.
- *Other aspects of physical examination of obesity*: A number of other factors in the physical examination may be utilized to help identify specific causes of the individual circumstance. For example, Cushing's syndrome with its striae, obesity, and hypertension is a result of increased levels of adrenal steroids [10]. Polycystic ovary disease is a common cause of obesity in younger women and is associated with excessive androgen and marked insulin resistance [11].

A number of genetic diseases may also cause obesity. Most common among these is Prader-Willi syndrome that includes hypertonia,

TABLE 4.2
Body Mass Index (BMI) (Using Either Pounds and Inches or Kilograms and Centimeters)

Body Mass Index (kg/m²)

Inches	19	20	21	22	23	24	25	26	27	28	29	30	31	32	33	34	35	36	37	38	39	40	Cm
58	91	95	100	105	110	115	119	124	129	134	138	143	148	153	158	162	167	172	177	181	186	191	
	41	43	45	48	50	52	54	56	58	61	63	65	67	69	71	73	76	78	80	82	84	86	147
59	94	99	104	109	114	119	124	128	133	138	143	148	153	158	163	168	173	178	183	188	193	198	
	43	45	47	50	52	54	56	59	61	63	65	68	70	72	74	77	79	81	83	86	88	90	150
60	97	102	107	112	118	123	128	133	138	143	148	153	158	164	169	174	179	184	189	194	199	204	
	44	46	49	51	53	55	58	60	62	65	67	69	72	74	76	79	81	83	85	88	90	92	152
61	100	106	111	116	121	127	132	137	143	148	153	158	164	169	174	180	185	190	195	201	206	211	
	46	48	50	53	55	58	60	62	65	67	70	72	74	76	79	82	84	86	89	91	94	96	155
62	104	109	115	120	125	131	136	142	147	153	158	164	169	175	180	186	191	196	202	207	213	218	
	47	50	52	55	57	60	62	65	67	70	72	75	77	80	82	85	87	90	92	95	97	100	158
63	107	113	118	124	130	135	141	146	152	158	163	169	175	180	186	192	197	203	208	214	220	225	
	49	51	54	56	59	61	64	67	69	72	74	77	79	82	84	87	90	92	95	97	100	102	160
64	110	116	122	128	134	140	145	151	157	163	169	174	180	186	192	198	203	209	215	221	227	233	
	50	52	55	58	60	63	66	68	71	73	76	79	81	84	87	89	92	94	97	100	102	105	162
65	114	120	126	132	138	144	150	156	162	168	174	180	186	192	198	204	210	216	222	228	234	240	
	52	54	57	60	63	65	68	71	74	76	79	82	84	87	90	93	95	98	101	103	106	109	165
66	117	124	130	136	142	148	155	161	167	173	179	185	191	198	204	210	216	223	229	235	241	247	
	54	56	59	62	65	68	71	73	76	79	82	85	87	90	93	96	99	102	104	107	110	113	168
67	121	127	134	140	147	153	159	166	172	178	185	191	198	204	210	217	223	229	236	242	248	255	
	55	58	61	64	66	69	72	75	78	81	84	87	90	92	95	98	101	104	107	110	113	116	170
68	125	131	138	144	151	158	164	171	177	184	190	197	203	210	217	223	230	236	243	249	256	263	
	57	60	63	66	69	72	75	78	81	84	87	90	93	96	99	102	105	108	111	114	117	120	173
69	128	135	142	149	155	162	169	176	182	189	196	203	209	216	223	230	237	243	250	257	264	270	
	58	61	64	67	70	74	77	80	83	86	89	92	95	98	101	104	107	110	113	116	119	123	175

(Continued)

TABLE 4.2 (Continued)
Body Mass Index (BMI) (Using Either Pounds and Inches or Kilograms and Centimeters)

Body Mass Index (kg/m²)

Inches	19	20	21	22	23	24	25	26	27	28	29	30	31	32	33	34	35	36	37	38	39	40	
70	132	139	146	153	160	167	174	181	188	195	202	209	216	223	230	236	243	250	257	264	271	278	
	60	63	67	70	73	76	79	82	86	89	92	95	98	101	105	108	111	114	117	120	124	127	178
71	136	143	150	157	165	172	179	186	193	200	207	215	222	229	236	243	250	258	265	272	279	286	
	62	65	68	71	75	78	81	84	87	91	94	97	100	104	107	110	113	117	120	123	126	130	180
72	140	147	155	162	169	177	184	191	199	206	213	221	228	235	243	250	258	265	272	280	287	294	
	64	67	70	74	77	80	84	87	90	94	97	100	104	107	111	114	117	121	124	127	131	134	183
73	144	151	159	166	174	182	189	197	204	212	219	227	234	242	250	257	265	272	280	287	295	303	
	65	68	72	75	79	82	86	89	92	96	99	103	106	110	113	116	120	123	127	130	133	137	185
74	148	155	163	171	179	187	194	202	210	218	225	233	241	249	256	264	272	280	288	295	303	311	
	67	71	74	78	81	85	88	92	95	99	102	106	110	113	117	120	124	127	131	134	138	141	188
75	152	160	168	176	184	192	200	208	216	224	232	240	247	255	263	271	279	287	295	303	311	319	
	69	72	76	79	83	87	90	94	97	101	105	108	112	116	119	123	126	130	134	137	141	144	190
76	156	164	172	180	189	197	205	213	221	230	238	246	254	262	271	279	287	295	303	312	320	328	
	71	74	78	82	86	89	93	97	101	104	108	112	115	119	123	127	130	134	138	142	145	149	193
BMI	19	20	21	22	23	24	25	26	27	28	29	30	31	32	33	34	35	36	37	38	39	40	BMI

Bray G: Identification, evaluation and treatment of obesity. In Rippe JM, Angelopoulos TJ. *Obesity Prevention and Treatment*, CRC Press (Boca Raton), 2012. Reprinted from *Obesity Prevention and Treatment* by Rippe J, Angelopoulos J, Angelopoulos T. Obesity and Heart Disease. In Rippe JM and Angelopoulos TA (eds) CRC Press (Boca Raton, FL), 2012. Used with permission of the Editor, James M. Rippe, MD.

Note: The body mass index is shown as *bold underlined* numbers at the top and bottom. To determine your BMI, select your height in either inches or centimeters and move across the row until you find your weight in pounds or inches. Your BMI can be read at the top or bottom.

The italics are for pounds and inches; **the bold is for kilograms and centimeters.**

Copyright 1999 George A. Bray

TABLE 4.3

Classification of Overweight and Obesity as Recommended by the National Heart, Lung, and Blood Institute Guidelines

Disease Risk[a] Relative to Normal Weight and Waist Circumference

			Waist Circumference	
	BMI (kg/m²)	Obesity Class	<102 cm (Men) <88 cm (Women)	>102 cm (Men) >88 cm (Women)
Underweight	<18.5		–	–
Normal[b]	18.5–24.9		–	–
Overweight	25.0–29.9		Increased	High
Obesity	30.0–34.9	1	High	Very high
	35.0–39.9	2	Very high	Very high
Extreme obesity	≥40.0	3	Extremely high	Extremely high

Bray G: Identification, evaluation and treatment of obesity. In Rippe JM, Angelopoulos TJ. *Obesity Prevention and Treatment*, CRC Press (Boca Raton), 2012. Reprinted from *Obesity Prevention and Treatment* by Rippe JM and Angelopoulos, TJ. Used with permission of the Editor, Dr. James M. Rippe. BMI, body mass index.

[a] Disease risk for type 2 diabetes, hypertension and cardiovascular disease.

[b] Increased waist can also be a marker for increased risk in normal weight individuals.

mental retardation, and sexual immaturity and can usually be recognized clinically. Although 40 other genetic causes have been associated with obesity, they only contribute to a small fraction of individuals who are obese.

- *Information from laboratory tests*: The third part of the evaluation comes from laboratory tests. These often come in "batteries" which may include a larger number of tests that may be needed, but unbundling these tests is usually more expensive than simply utilizing the bundle. The most important tests in these bundles include the following:
  - *Plasma glucose*: Since over 9% of the adult population has diabetes, it is important to measure fasting blood glucose. If the question of diabetes or glucose intolerance is indicated, further testing including hemoglobin A1C would be appropriate. (See also Chapter 13.)
  - *Plasma lipids*: A low level of HDL cholesterol and high triglyceride levels are both important for the diagnosis of metabolic syndrome and are both parts of significant lipid abnormalities which increase the risk of heart disease [12].
  - *Thyroid-stimulating hormone*: Thyroid-stimulating hormone (TSH) is important as an index of hypothyroidism. This can occur in up to 4% of older women and may be a factor in weight gain in these individuals.
  - *Prostate-specific androgens*: Prostate cancer is one of the male cancers associated with obesity. PSA is a common screening test in men. The

relationship between obesity and prostate cancer highlights its value in screening overweight men.

- *Specialized tests*: Given the relationship of obesity to multiple other metabolic conditions, other specialized tests may be obtained including the following:
  - *Sleep study*: (useful in demonstrating obstructive sleep apnea which is common in obesity)
  - *Ultrasound of the gallbladder*: There is a high prevalence of gallstones in obese men and women. This test may be useful if there are any complaints of indigestion [13].
  - *Electrocardiogram and echocardiogram*: EKG is a common part of regular physical examination. EKG may be difficult to interpret in an individual with obesity. Echocardiography may be indicated due to the multiple interactions between obesity and heart disease. (See also Chapter 12.)
  - *Mammography*: Mammography since breast cancer is increased in women with obesity. Mammography is part of regular physical examinations of women, particularly those over the age of 40. (See also Chapter 15.)
- *Tests for Metabolic syndrome*: Metabolic syndrome is a complex of traits associated with increased risk of both CVD and T2DM. A variety of different criteria are available for the determination of metabolic syndrome [12]. Features utilized in the National Cholesterol Education Program are found in Table 4.4.

  Metabolic syndrome is very common and highly associated with obesity. It has been estimated that 36%–38% of the adult population in the

---

TABLE 4.4

Clinical Features of the Metabolic Syndrome

Risk Factor	Defining Level
Abdominal obesity (waist circumference)	
Men	>102 cm (>40 in)
Women	>88 cm (>35 in)
HDL cholesterol	
Men	<40 mg/dl
Women	<50 mg/dl
Triglycerides	>150 mg/dl
Fasting glucose	>100 mg/dl
Blood pressure (systolic/diastolic)	>130 mmHg/>85 mmHg

Bray G: Identification, evaluation and treatment of obesity. In Rippe JM, Angelopoulos TJ. *Obesity Prevention and Treatment*, CRC Press (Boca Raton), 2012. Used with permission of the Editor Dr. James M. Rippe. HDL, high density lipoprotein.

United States has metabolic syndrome depending on the criteria utilized. Metabolic syndrome is one of the most under-diagnosed conditions in clinical practice, so making the measurements necessary to determine if metabolic syndrome is present and counseling patients about the risk factors associated with metabolic syndrome represent an important area of clinical counseling and measurement. (See also Chapter 14.)

4.4   GUIDELINES FOR TREATMENT

Following the history, physical examination, and laboratory data, the risk factors associated with elevated BMI, fat distribution, and weight gain the level of physical activity can be evaluated and put in context. Several algorithms have been developed for this purpose. A very effective one was developed by the NHLBI. This is found in Figure 4.1

It should be noted that even individuals who are in the healthy weight category of a BMI between 20 and 25 may become individuals with obesity by the ages of 60–69. The Women's Health Study also showed that individuals with a BMI>23 start to substantially increase their risk of heart disease [13].

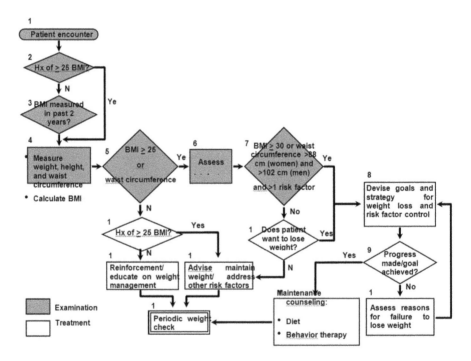

FIGURE 4.1 Treatment algorithm from the National Heart, Lung, and Blood Institute. (BMI, body mass index; Hx, History. From U.S. Department of Health and Human Services Public Health Service National Institutes of Health National Heart, Lung, and Blood Institute NIH Publication No. 00-4084. Adapted by Bray G: Identification, evaluation and treatment of obesity. In Rippe JM, Angelopoulos TJ. *Obesity Prevention and Treatment*, CRC Press (Boca Raton), 2012. Used with permission of the Editor Dr. James M. Rippe.)

Questions to consider before initiating therapy for obesity.

- *Is the patient ready to lose weight?*: It is important, before starting any treatment, to ascertain whether or not the patient is truly ready to make changes. One series of questions developed by Brownell et al. is entitled "The Dietary Readiness Test" [14]. This can be utilized to assess readiness to change. It is also important, when starting a weight loss program, to accommodate individual needs such as ethnic factors, age, and other differences. The approach to clinical decision-making must be utilized with flexibility. Since a variety of treatments are available, it may be useful to select treatments based on BMI. Table 4.5 provides some guidance in this area.
- *Do patient and doctor have realistic expectations?*: It is important to frame the issue of weight loss and why it is important to the patient. One survey showed that only 40% of clinicians ever discuss the importance of weight loss with their patients [15]. Furthermore, many patients have unrealistic expectations of how much weight they would like to lose or if it is even possible to lose [16]. In one study, patients were asked about how much weight they would like to lose to achieve their dream weight. Their responses indicated their goal was an average of 38% below their current levels. Nearly half of individuals who lose weight achieve a weight outcome that they describe as either "disappointing" or "severely disappointing."

  An initial weight loss goal of 5%–7% can be achieved by most patients and will improve many of the risk factors associated with obesity. This was demonstrated both in the Diabetes Prevention Program [17] and the Look AHEAD Trial [18]. It should also be carefully explained to patients that hitting a "plateau" is common during weight loss and that if individuals carefully examine both their nutritional and physical activity choices, they can break through this plateau. It should also be emphasized to overweight or obese individuals that this condition is a chronic one and will require lifelong vigilance.
- *Quality of Life*: Quality of life is, of course, important to all patients [19]. This affects many different areas from day-to-day functioning as well as a reduction in comorbidities which can significantly be improved with weight

TABLE 4.5

Selection of Treatments Based on the Body Mass Index

Treatment	25–29.9	27–29.9	30–34.9	35–39.9	>40
Diet, exercise, lifestyle	+	+	+	+	+
Pharmacotherapy		With co-morbidities	+	+	+
Surgery				With co-morbidties	+

Bray G: Identification, evaluation and treatment of obesity. In Rippe JM, Angelopoulos TJ. *Obesity Prevention and Treatment*, CRC Press (Boca Raton), 2012. Used with permission from the Editor Dr. James M. Rippe.

loss. Weight loss can also reduce wear and tear on joints and, thereby, slow the development of arthritis. Sleep apnea usually also resolves with weight loss which can create less daytime drowsiness and increased energy. Psychological improvement is also often achieved. Loss of 5% or more or initial weight almost always translates into improved mobility, increased exercise tolerance, and heightened self-esteem. Clinicians should focus on all of these multiple benefits of weight loss which will improve quality of life.

4.5 GUIDELINES FOR TREATMENT BY AGE GROUP

One way of grouping treatments by age group has been supplied by prominent weight loss researcher Dr. George Bray [20]. He has divided a strategy into age groups, starting with age 1–10, followed by ages 11–50, and then 51 and higher. These strategies are outlined in Tables 4.6–4.8. (Reprinted from *Obesity Prevention and Treatment* by Rippe JM and Angelopoulos, TJ with permission of the editors.)

4.6 SUMMARY/CONCLUSIONS

Given the prevalence of overweight and obesity as well as the association between obesity and multiple, serious comorbid conditions, it is important that all clinicians have a structured approach to counsel individuals concerning the prevention and treatment of obesity. The evaluation of the patient who is overweight or obese starts with obtaining a clinical history based on when weight gain occurred and any other associated conditions. This is followed by an obesity-focused physical examination and information from laboratory tests. In some instances, specialized tests will also be required.

TABLE 4.6
Therapeutic Strategies: Age 1–10 Years

	Therapeutic Strategies		
Predictors of Overweight	Pre-overweight at Risk	Preclinical Overweight	Clinical Overweight
Positive family history	Family counseling	Family behavior therapy	Treat co-morbidities
Genetic defects	Reduce inactivity	Exercise	Exercise
(dysmorphic)		Low-fat/low-energy-	Low-fat/low-energy-
Prader-Willi syndrome		dense diet	dense diet
(Bardet-Biedl; Cohen)			
Hypothalamic injury			
Low metabolic rate			
Diabetic mother			

Bray G: Identification, evaluation and treatment of obesity. In Rippe JM, Angelopoulos TJ. *Obesity Prevention and Treatment*, CRC Press (Boca Raton), 2012.Used with permission of the Editor Dr. James M. Rippe.

TABLE 4.7

Therapeutic Strategies: Appropriate for Individuals from Age 11–50

	Therapeutic Strategies		
Predictors of Overweight	**Preoverweight at Risk**	**Preclinical Overweight**	**Clinical Overweight**
Positive family history of diabetes or obesity	Reduce sedentary lifestyle	Behavior therapy	Treat co-morbidities
Endocrine disorders (polycystic ovary syndrome)	Low-fat/low-energy-dense diet	Low-fat/low-energy-dense diet	Drug treatment for overweight
Multiple pregnancies	Portion control	Reduce sedentary lifestyle	Reduce sedentary lifestyle
Marriage			Low-fat/low-energy-dense diet
Smoking cessation			Behavior therapy
Medication			Surgery

Bray G: Identification, evaluation and treatment of obesity. In Rippe JM, Angelopoulos TJ. *Obesity Prevention and Treatment*, CRC Press (Boca Raton), 2012. Used with permission of the Editor Dr. James M. Rippe.

TABLE 4.8

Therapeutic Strategies: Appropriate for Individuals over 51 Years of Age

Predictors of Overweight	Therapeutic Strategies		
	Preoverweight at Risk	**Preclinical Overweight**	**Clinical Overweight**
Menopause	Few individuals remain in this subgroup	Behavior therapy	Treat co-morbidities
Declining growth hormone		Low-fat/low-energy-dense diet	Drug treatment for overweight
Declining testosterone		Reduce sedentary lifestyle	Reduce sedentary lifestyle
Smoking cessation			Low-fat/low-energy-dense diet
Medication			Behavior therapy
			Surgery

Bray G: Identification, evaluation and treatment of obesity. In Rippe JM, Angelopoulos TJ. *Obesity Prevention and Treatment*, CRC Press (Boca Raton), 2012. Used with permission of the Editor Dr. James M. Rippe.

It is also of paramount importance that the patient is ready to lose weight and that realistic expectations are maintained by both the patient and the physician. Numerous trials including such large studies as the Diabetes Prevention Program and the Look AHEAD Trial have demonstrated that multiple risk factors for chronic disease may be improved by a weight loss of 5%–7% of initial body weight. These amounts of weight may be smaller than patients initially hope to achieve. However, from a medical standpoint, they represent good initial goals that can significantly improve the health of virtually every patient. It should also be noted that even individuals in the "healthy" weight range with a BMI between 20 and 25 may experience weight gain and/or obesity by the time they are in their 60 s. Thus, the issue of weight and health should be discussed with every patient.

CLINICAL APPLICATIONS

- Both adult weight gain and overweight and obesity are associated with increased risk of various chronic conditions including heart disease, diabetes, and cancer.
- A targeted approach to physical examination and history and laboratory values focused on specific issues related to overweight and obesity should be followed.
- A useful algorithm from the NHLBI can help the clinician work his/her way through a comprehensive evaluation of obesity.

REFERENCES

1. Bray G.A. *A Guide of Obesity and the Metabolic Syndrome.* New York: Taylor Francis, 2011.
2. Klein S., Burke L., Bray G., et al. American Heart Association Council on Nutrition, Physical Activity, and Metabolism. Clinical implications of obesity with specific focus on cardiovascular disease: A statement for professionals from the American Heart Association Council on Nutrition, Physical Activity, and Metabolism: endorsed by the American College of Cardiology Foundation. *Circulation.* 2004;110:2952–67.
3. National Institutes of Health, National Heart, Lung, and Blood Institute, North American Association for the Study of Obesity. The Practical Guide. Identification, Evaluation, and Treatment of Overweight and Obesity in Adults. Bethesda: National Institutes of Health, October 2000: NIH Publication Number 00-4084.
4. NHLBI Obesity Education Initiative Expert Panel on the Identification, Evaluation, and Treatment of Overweight and Obesity in Adults. Clinical guidelines on the identification, evaluation, and treatment of overweight and obesity in adults—The evidence report. *Obes Res.* 1998;6(Suppl 2): 51S–209S.
5. Obesity: preventing and managing the global epidemic. Report of a WHO consultation. World Health Organ Tech Rep Ser 894: i-xii, 1–253.
6. Despres J.P. Dyslipidaemia and obesity. *Bailliere Clinic Endo Metab.* 1994;8(629):660.
7. Despres J.P., Abdominal obesity as important component of insulin-resistance syndrome. *Nutrition.* 1993;4:452–459.
8. US Department of Health and Human Services: Body measurements. In: *Clinician's Handbook of Preventive Services: Put Prevention into Family Practice.* 1994; pp. 141–146.
9. Roche A., Heymsfield S.B., Lohman T. *Human Body Composition.* Champaign, IL: Human Kinetics, 1996.
10. Arnaldi G., Angeli A., Atkinson A., et al. Diagnosis and complications of Cushing's syndrome: A consensus statement. *J Clin Endocrinol Metab.* 2003;88(12):5593–602.
11. Welt K., Gudmundsson A., Arason G., et al. Characterizing discrete subsets of polycystic ovary syndrome as defined by the Rotterdam criteria: The impact of weight on phenotype and metabolic features. *J Clin Endocrinol Metab.* 2006;91(12):4842–8.
12. Expert Panel on Detection, Evaluation, and Treatment of High Blood Cholesterol in Adults. Executive summary of the third report of the national cholesterol education

program (NCEP) Expert panel on detection, evaluation, and treatment of high blood cholesterol in adults (Adult Treatment Panel III). *JAMA*. 2001;285(19):2486–97.

13. Nurses' Health Study, Bassuk S.S., Manson J.E. Lifestyle and risk of cardiovascular disease and type 2 diabetes in women: A review of the epidemiologic evidence. *Am J Lifestyle Med*. 2008;2(3):191–213.

14. Brownell K. Dieting readiness. *Weight Control Digest*. 1990;1:1–9.

15. Galuska A., Will C., Serdula K., et al. Are health care professionals advising obese patients to lose weight? *JAMA*. 1999;282(16):1576–1578.

16. Foster D., Wadden A., Vogt A., et al. What is a reasonable weight loss? Patients' expectations and evaluations of obesity treatment outcomes. *J Consult Clin Psychol*. 1997;65(1):79–85.

17. The Diabetes Prevention Program Research Group. The diabetes prevention program (DPP): Description of lifestyle intervention. *Diabetes Care*. 2002;25:2165–2171.

18. Look AHEAD Research Group, Wing R.R., Bolin P., et al. Cardiovascular effects of intensive lifestyle intervention in type 2 diabetes. *N Engl J Med*. 2013;369:145–54.

19. Rippe J., Price J., Hess S., Kline G., DeMers K., Damitz S., Kreidieh I., Freedson, P. Improved psychological well being, quality of life and health practices in moderately overweight women participating in a 12 week structured weight loss program. *Obesity Research*. 1998;6:208–218.

20. Bray G. Identification, evaluation and treatment of obesity. In Rippe J.M., Angelopoulos T.J. (eds.) *Obesity Prevention and Treatment*. Boca Raton, FL: CRC Press, 2012.

5 Exercise Management for the Patient with Obesity

James M. Rippe, MD

Rippe Lifestyle Institute
University of Massachusetts Medical School

CONTENTS

5.1 INTRODUCTION

Overweight and obesity are significant public health problems in the United States and around the world [1]. In the United States, the prevalence of overweight, obesity, and severe obesity are approximately 73.6%, 42.5%, and 9%, respectively [2]. These high prevalence rates raise significant public health questions since excess body weight is associated with many other chronic diseases, including cardiovascular disease (CVD), type 2 diabetes (T2DM), some forms of cancer, musculoskeletal disorder, and many others [3,4]. (See also Chapters 12–16).

Interventions that are cost effective are needed to prevent overweight and obesity and also to help reduce the likelihood of weight gain. Lifestyle factors are essential to these approaches to contribute optimum energy balance to prevent weight gain or energy imbalance resulting in energy deficit to promote weight loss. One of the key lifestyle factors implicated in these prevention and treatment strategies is physical activity [5].

5.2 THE EFFECT OF PHYSICAL ACTIVITY ON PREVENTION OF WEIGHT GAIN

Many efforts in the area of overweight and obesity in adults are focused on the treatment of weight loss. However, it is also vitally important to consider effective approaches to prevent weight gain to reduce the prevalence of overweight and obesity in the first place. Physical activity may be an important lifestyle behavior

DOI: 10.1201/9781003099116-6

that can contribute to these prevention efforts. There is considerable evidence to support the influence of physical activity on the prevention of weight gain. These include cross-sectional studies which have supported an inverse relationship between physical activity and both BMI and body fat measures [6–12]. There are also prospective data from the NHANES-1 Epidemiologic Follow-up Study [13], the Aerobic Center for Longitudinal Studies [14], Women's Health Study [15], and the Harvard Alumni Study [16] to support the importance of physical activity of the prevention of weight gain.

It appears that the amount of physical activity necessary to prevent weight gain of at least 3% of current body weight is somewhere between 150 and 250 minutes per week. While this may seem daunting for many individuals, it only increases the recommendations from the Physical Activity Guidelines for Americans 2018 (PAGA 2018) by 100 minutes per week. The PAGA 2018 recommended that all adults should try to accumulate 150 minutes of moderate intensity physical activity per week [17]. Furthermore, regular physical activity may be quite helpful in retaining lean body mass and may play a role in lowering weight gain following significant weight loss.

5.3   EFFECTS OF PHYSICAL ACTIVITY ON WEIGHT LOSS

- *Cardiovascular activity*: The effects of physical activity on weight loss when not coupled with a concurrent reduction in energy intake appear to be modest. In several studies, a weight loss averaging between 1% and 2% in studies lasting between 6 and 18 months has been reported [18]. The amount of weight loss due solely to exercise may be dose related. The American College of Sports Medicine (ACSM) concluded that there was no significant change in body weight in response to <150 minutes per week of physical activity [19]. Whereas 2–3 kg of weight loss was observed with active >150 minutes per week and 5–7.5 kg for amounts between 225 and 420 minutes per week of moderate intensity physical activity.

- *Resistance exercise*: Less information is available related to resistance exercise and weight management, particularly in the absence of aerobic forms of physical activity. It has been suggested that resistance exercise may increase lean body mass, thereby enhancing metabolism and influencing body weight [19]. The systematic reviews in this area, however, have concluded that resistance exercise in the absence of energy restriction results in modest weight loss [20]. It may be argued, however, that increases in lean muscle mass may mask decreases in body fat. In addition, there is some suggestion that resistance exercise may result in significant reductions of total body mass and, in particular, subcutaneous abdominal adiposity. This is an area of active research.

- *Lifestyle activity*: Numerous organizations including the PAGA 2018 Scientific Report as well as ACSM have recommended non-structured forms of physical activity as a means to increase energy expenditure [19]. Many of these studies have used pedometers with the recommendation that patients increase the number of steps walked. These findings have typically been more prevalent in research regarding physical activity. In one study, an increase of 2,100 steps per day resulted in a modest decrease of weight loss of 2–3 kg. The area of research involving increases in step counts and weight management suggests that 10,000 steps per day with a third of them as part of a moderate to vigorous intensity physical activity strategy appears to be most successful in terms of weight loss. This is equivalent to approximately five miles of walking per day.

- *Sedentary behavior*: Sedentary behavior has been shown in numerous studies to correlate with multiple chronic diseases. The PAGA 2018 Guidelines explored the relationship between sedentary behavior and indices of obesity. In systematic reviews in this area, limited evidence was found that sedentary behavior was associated with weight gain or other indices of overweight or obesity [20,21]. Nonetheless, there is a robust literature relating to sedentary behavior and increased risk of both cardiovascular disease (CVD) and T2DM. It would appear that sedentary behavior must be combined with either light intensity or moderate intensity physical activity in order to result in weight loss.
- *Duration of physical activity bouts*: A number of reports including the 1995 Report from the Physical Activity Centers for Disease Control and Prevention (CDC) and the American College of Sports Medicine (ACSM) suggested that physical activity needed to be 8–10 minutes in duration per session to result in benefits [22]. However, since that time, studies that have examined physical activity in lesser amounts of per bout and have concluded that even lesser duration bouts of physical activity result in multiple benefits. This was the conclusion of the PAGA 2018 Scientific Report. It should be pointed out, however, that these shorter bouts of physical activity may not result in weight loss. It would appear that bouts of physical activity that are at least 10 minutes in duration still are more desirable if the goal is weight loss.
- *Physical activity combined with reduction in energy intake*: The most common form of weight loss recommendation involves physical activity in combination with a reduction in energy intake. In this area, physical activity can add 2–3 kg of weight loss beyond what is achieved by an energy-restricted diet alone. In one study, it was determined that 200–300 minutes of moderate intensity physical activity per week showed improved weight loss at 18 months as a component of a comprehensive behavioral weight loss prevention.
- *Role of physical activity in surgically induced weight loss*: Bariatric surgery is an effective method for the treatment of obesity. Recommendations for bariatric surgery typically include BMI > 30 within the context of established comorbidities such as CVD or T2DM or BMI > 40 kg/m^2. Unfortunately, few patients following bariatric surgery participate in regular physical activity, although several studies have shown that weight loss following the initial weight loss from bariatric surgery is enhanced by physical activity ≥80–150 minutes of moderate intensity physical activity per week as recommended by the PAGA 2018.

5.4 WEIGHT LOSS VARIABILITY IN RESPONSE TO PHYSICAL ACTIVITY

Researchers in weight loss have often observed considerable inter-individual invariability in weight loss in response to physical activity. It is possible that physical activity may result in more weight loss in some individuals than others or that similar amounts of physical activity in weight loss may occur between individuals who have similar doses of physical activity. In one study on weight loss in response to highly controlled exercise, weight loss in a range of approximately 3.0–12.0 kg was reported. A number of factors may contribute to variability in weight in response to physical activity.

- *Biological factors*: There may be biological factors that contribute to weight loss observed in response to physical activity. Bouchard et al. studied seven pairs of identical twins examined over a period of 93 days, while energy intake was held constant and physical activity performed twice a day [23]. Subjects were also monitored 24 hours a day to attempt to control and minimize any variability in managing energy intake or physical activity. The results of this study demonstrated weight loss was similar within each pair of twins but highly variable between pairs of twins. Thus, there may be biological underpinnings to weight loss variability.
- *Influence of physical activity on other components of energy expenditure*: Negative energy balance is essential to weight loss. Physical activity is the largest and most variable component of energy expenditure [24]. Moreover, it has been suggested that physical activity may influence other components of energy expenditure such as resting metabolic rate (RMR) which can further affect full energy consumption. There may be both acute and chronic increases in RMR in response to physical activity [25]. This is particularly important for individuals who are obese since RMR tends to decrease during weight loss which can result in a decrease in total energy expenditure and adversely impact weight loss maintenance [26]. Even with physical activity, RMR may decrease. Nonetheless, physical activity is very important on multiple levels for both weight loss and maintenance of weight loss.
- *Influence of physical activity on energy intake*: There is also evidence of considerable inter-individual variability in energy intake in response to physical activity. In one study of physical activity and weight loss, positive increase in energy consumption occurred in 15% of study subjects. In another study, 58% of participants consumed more calories following a 35–45 minute period of activity compared to a seated rest period [27]. These data suggest that for some patients who are obese physical activity increases hunger and appetite, while in others physical activity may enhance satiety, both of which can impact energy intake.
- *Factors influencing adherence to physical activity*: The variability of weight loss may also reflect an individual's ability to adopt and adhere to an adequate dose of physical activity to promote weight loss. In one study, there was a strong correlation between high levels of physical activity and

self-efficacy [28]. The issue of self-efficacy has been established as strongly correlated with lifestyle changes in a variety of areas. (See Chapter 7.) This suggests that individuals prescribing physical activity for weight loss should be trained in areas of behavioral change in order to effectively prescribe physical activity as a component to weight loss.

5.5 PHYSICAL ACTIVITY, FITNESS, AND HEALTH OUTCOMES

Multiple other benefits can come from physical activity in addition to weight loss in individuals who are overweight and obese. A number of studies have shown that cardiorespiratory fitness improves only if physical activity is included as a component of the intervention program. These benefits occur whether or not the intervention results in weight loss [29]. It should be noted that fitness does not improve significantly when weight loss is induced by energy restriction alone. The magnitude of improvement in cardiorespiratory fitness depends on the dose of physical activity performed. This dose/response relationship has been found in multiple areas including weight loss and obesity and is important in areas such as quality of life and reduction of risk or chronic diseases associated with obesity.

- *Effects on mortality*: The level of cardiorespiratory fitness and reduced mortality is present in obese individuals even when adjusted for the level of adiposity. This has led to the debate which has often been characterized as "fit versus fat." Nonetheless, higher levels of cardiorespiratory fitness do not completely ameliorate the risk of high levels of BMI or body fatness. This has been demonstrated in a number of studies including the Lipid Research Clinic Study [30] and the Look AHEAD Trial [31]. In the Look AHEAD Trial in patients with T2DM who achieved a weight loss of only 10% after 1 year achieved a 20% reduction in the primary outcome of cardiovascular disease. Fitness, however, was not associated with this outcome. However, an increase of ≥ 2 METs in aerobic capacity was associated with a 23% reduction in secondary outcomes such as coronary artery bypass grafting, carotid endarterectomy percutaneous coronary intervention, admission to hospital for congestive heart failure, and total mortality. Taken together, these findings suggest that interventions for patients who are overweight or obese should focus on both weight loss and improving fitness to elicit risk reduction and of all cause cardiovascular disease mortality.
- *Effects of risk factors on cardiovascular disease*: Cardiorespiratory fitness appears to partially contribute to reduction in cardiovascular disease mortality in patients who are overweight or obese. This may be the result of the influence of cardiorespiratory fitness on risk factors known to be associated with cardiovascular disease such as elevated blood pressure, lipids, and inflammatory biomarkers, as well as T2DM. It should be noted that fitness may not completely eliminate the association between adiposity and these risk factors for cardiovascular disease.
  - *Blood pressure*: Hypertension is a significant risk factor for CVD. Both fitness and fatness appear to have an impact on blood pressure in

individuals who are obese. Findings from several studies suggest both BMI and fitness may be important for blood pressure control in individuals who are overweight or obese and that both should be targets of clinical interventions [32]. Regular aerobic activity in individuals who are overweight or obese, as well as normal weight individuals, has been demonstrated to reduce both systolic and diastolic blood pressure between 2 and 3 mmHg. (See also Chapter 12.)

- *Lipids*: Dyslipidemia is considered a primary risk for cardiovascular disease. Interventions that target obesity may have a favorable effect on blood lipids. However, physical activity appears to have a very modest influence on blood lipids in individuals who are overweight or obese. In a meta-analysis of studies that included adults who are overweight or obese total cholesterol was reduced by 3.4 mg/dl, LDL was reduced by 3.0 mg/dl and HDL was increased by 1.6 mg/dl in response to physical activity interventions that did not include dietary restriction or result in significant weight loss [33]. In this same study, triglycerides were reported to be reduced by an average of 16.1 mg/dl. When physical activity is added to caloric restriction, the CALERIE Study showed significant reductions in both total cholesterol and LDL. These improvements were not observed when calorie restriction alone was studied, which did not include physical activity as part of the intervention.

- *Inflammatory markers*: It has been suggested that overweight and obesity result in total body inflammation. C-reactive protein (CRP), interlukin-6 (IL-6), tumor necrosis factor-alpha (TNFα), and the anti-inflammatory molecule, adiponectin contribute to the process of atherosclerosis [34]. It has been suggested that increased physical activity might improve these inflammatory markers. However, several studies have reported no association between cardiorespiratory fitness and measures of inflammation [35,36].

5.6   SUMMARY/CONCLUSIONS

Physical activity can play an important role in the management of individuals who are overweight or obese. In particular, physical activity decreases the likelihood of weight gain and the incidence of obesity. Physical activity results in only modest weight loss on the order of 0.5–3.0 kg in trials of up to 6 months. When physical activity is combined with a reduction in energy intake, physical activity can enhance weight loss by approximately 20% beyond the magnitude of weight loss achieved through reduced energy intake alone. Moreover, physical activity can result in a reduction in risk of both CVD and T2DM irrespective of whether or not it contributes to weight loss. For all these reasons, regular physical activity should be considered to be an integral and important component of overall prescriptions for individuals who are overweight or obese for either weight loss or general health considerations.

PRACTICAL APPLICATIONS

- Clinicians should include physical activity as a component of therapeutic regimens both for decreasing the likelihood of weight gain and also for decreasing obesity.
- Physical activity alone results in only modest short-term weight loss. However, it is critically important as a component of long-term maintenance of weight loss.
- For all of these reasons, clinicians should emphasize the need for patients to engage in a sufficient amount of physical activity both for prevention of weight gain or if overweight already as a component of weight loss.
- At least 150 minutes of moderate to vigorous intensity physical activity per week appears to be necessary in order to make significant contributions to weight loss. This is consistent with the physical activity recommendations from the recently released Physical Activity Guidelines for Americans 2018 Scientific Report.

REFERENCES

1. Flegal K., Kruszon-Moran D., Carroll M., et al. Trends in obesity among adults in the United States, 2005 to 2014. *JAMA*. 2016;315: 2284–2291.
2. CDC: National Center for Health Statistics. Prevalence of Overweight, Obesity, and Severe Obesity Among Children and Adolescents Aged 2–19 Years: United States, 1963–1965 Through 2015–2016 by Fryar CD, Carroll MD, Ogden CL. Division of Health and Nutrition Examination Surveys. https://www.cdc.gov/nchs/data/hestat/obesity_child_15_16/obesity_child_15_16.pdf. Accessed January 2021.
3. Jensen M., Ryan D., Apovian C., et al. 2013 AHA/ACC/TOS guideline for the management of overweight and obesity in adults: A report of the American College of Cardiology/American Heart Association task force on practice guidelines and the obesity society. *J Am Coll Cardiol*. 2014;63: 2985–3023.
4. National Institutes of Health National Heart Lung and Blood Institute. Clinical guidelines on the identification, evaluation, and treatment of overweight and obesity in adults: The evidence report. *Obes Res*. 1998;6(suppl.2): 51S–209S.
5. Jakicic J., Rogers R., Davis K., et al. Role of physical activity and exercise in treating patients with overweight and obesity. *Clin Chem*. 2018;64(1): 99–107.
6. Cameron N., Nichols J., Hill L., et al. Associations between physical activity and BMI, body fatness, and visceral adiposity in overweight or obese Latino and non-Latino adults. *Int J Obes*. 2017;41: 873–877.
7. Fan J., Brown B., Hanson H., et al. Moderate to vigorous physical activity and weight outcomes: Does every minute count? *Am J Prev Med*. 2013;28: 41–49.
8. Glazer N., Lyass A., Esliger D., et al. Sustained and shorter bouts of physical activity are related to cardiovascular health. *Med Sci Sports Exerc*. 2013;45: 109–115.
9. Jakicic J., Gregg E., Knowler W., et al. Physical activity patterns of overweight and obese individuals with type 2 diabetes in the Look AHEAD Study. *Med Sci Sports Exerc*. 2010;42: 1995–2005.
10. Jefferis B., Parsons T., Sartini C., et al. Does duration of physical activity bouts matter for adiposity and metabolic syndrome? A cross-sectional study of older British men. *Int J Behav Nutr Phys Act*. 2016;13: 36.

11. Loprinzi P., Cardinal B. Association between biologic outcomes and objectively measured physical activity accumulated in >10-minute bout and <10-minute bouts. *Am J Health Promot.* 2013;27: 143–151.
12. Wolff-Hughes D., Fitzhugh E., Bassett D., Total activity counts and bouted minutes of moderate-to-vigorous physical activity: Relationships with cardiometabolic biomarkers using 2003–2006 NHANES. *J Phys Act Health.* 2015;12: 694–700.
13. Williamson D., Madans J., Anda R., et al. Recreational physical activity and ten-year weight change in a US national cohort. *Int J Obes.* 1993;17: 279–286.
14. DiPietro L., Dziura J., Blair S. Estimated change in physical activity level (PAL) and prediction of 5-year weight change in men: The aerobics center longitudinal study. *Int J Obes.* 2004;28: 1541–1547.
15. Lee I., Djousse L., Sesso H., et al. Physical activity and weight gain prevention. *JAMA.* 2010;303: 1173–1179.
16. Shiroma E., Sesso H., Lee I. Physical activity and weight gain prevention in older men. *Int J Obes (Lond)* 2012;36: 1165–1169.
17. 2018 Physical Activity Guidelines Advisory Committee. 2018 Physical Activity Guidelines Advisory Committee Scientific Report. U.S. Department of Health and Human Services: Washington, DC, 2018.
18. Jakicic J., Otto A., Semler L., et al. Effect of physical activity on 18-month weight change in overweight adults. *Obesity.* 2011;19: 100–109.
19. Donnelly J., Blair S., Jakicic J., et al. ACSM Position Stand on appropriate intervention strategies for weight loss and prevention of weight regain for adults. *Med Sci Sports Exerc.* 2009;42: 459–471.
20. Donnelly J., Jakicic J., Pronk N., et al. Is resistance exercise effective for weight management? *Evid Based Prev Med.* 2004;1: 21–29.
21. Thorpe A., Own N., Neuhaus M., et al. Sedentary behaviors and subsequent health outcomes in adults: A systematic review of longitudinal studies. *Am J Prev Med* 2011;41: 207–215.
22. Pate R., Pratt M., Blair S., et al. Physical activity and public health: A recommendation from the Centers for Disease and Prevention and the American College of Sports Medicine. *JAMA.* 1995;273: 402–407.
23. Bouchard C., Tremblay A., Despres J., et al. The response to exercise with constant energy intake in identical twins. *Obes Res.* 1994;2: 400–410.
24. Ravussin E., Bogardus C. Relationship of genetics, age, and physical fitness to daily energy expenditure and fuel utilization. *Am J Clin Nutr.* 1989;49: 968–975.
25. Tremblay A., Fontaine E., Poehlman E., et al. The effect of exercise-training on resting metabolic rate in lean and moderately obese individuals. *Int J Obes.* 1986;10: 511–517.
26. Tremblay A. Physical activity level and resting metabolic rate. In: Bouchard C., Katzmarzyk P.T. (eds). *Physical Activity and Obesity.* Second Edition. Human Kinetics: Champaign, IL, 2010.
27. Finlayson G., Bryant E., Blundell J., et al. Acute compensatory eating following exercise is associated with implicit hedonic wanting for food. *Physiol Behav.* 2009;97: 62–67.
28. Gallagher K., Jakicic J., Napolitano M., et al. Psychosocial factors related to physical activity and weight loss in overweight women. *Med Sci Sports Exerc.* 2006;38: 971–980.
29. Ross R., Dagnone D., Jones P., Smith H., et al. Reduction in obesity and related comorbid conditions after diet-induced weight loss or exercise-induced weight loss in men. *Ann Intern Med.* 2000;133: 92–103.
30. Stevens J., Cai J., Evenson K., et al. Fitness and fatness as predictors of mortality from all causes and from cardiovascular disease in men and women in the lipid research clinics study. *Am J Epidemiol.* 2002;156: 832–841.
31. The Look AHEAD Research Group. Association of the magnitude of weight loss and changes in physical fitness with long-term cardiovascular disease outcomes in

overweight or obese people with type 2 diabetes: A post-hoc analysis of the Look AHEAD randomised clinical trial. *Lancet Diabetes Endocrinol.* 2016;4: 913–921.

32. Rankinen T., Church T., Rice T., et al. Cardiorespiratory fitness, BMI, and risk of hypertension: The Hypgene study. *Med Sci Sports Exerc.* 2007;39: 1687–1692.
33. Kelley G., Kelley K., Tran Z. Aerobic exercise, lipids and lipoproteins in overweight and obese adults: A meta-analysis of randomized controlled trials. *Int J Obes.* 2005;29: 881–893.
34. Van Gaal L., Mertens I., DeBlock C. Mechanisms linking obesity with cardiovascular disease. *Nature.* 2006;444: 875–880.
35. Church T., Earnest C., Thompson A., et al. Exercise without weight loss does not reduce C-reactive protein: The INFLAME study. *Med Sci Sports Exerc.* 2010;42: 708–716.
36. Nicklas B., Ambrosius W., Messier S., et al. Diet-induced weight loss, exercise, and chronic inflammation in older, obese adults: A randomized controlled clinical trial. *Am J Clin Nutr* 2004;79: 544–551.

6 Behavioral Management for the Patient with Obesity

John P. Foreyt, PhD
Baylor College of Medicine

CONTENTS

6.1 INTRODUCTION

Behavior modification is the foundation of long-term weight control programs for patients with obesity. The American Heart Association/American College of Cardiology/The Obesity Society Guideline recommends behavior modification for all patients receiving treatment for obesity [1]. Changes in diet and exercise remain the ultimate goal, but it is the behavioral strategies that help patients overcome the challenges of making the needed changes to achieve a healthier lifestyle.

For the health care provider to be most effective in helping patients make needed lifestyle changes, it is important to have a "toolbox" of strategies. Because no two patients are alike, the toolbox will help the provider tailor interventions to the unique needs of each patient. This chapter describes several strategies that have shown success in helping patients lose and maintain weight and achieve a healthier lifestyle. Because health care providers are busy and oftentimes do not have the time they would like to spend with each patient, we also summarize the critical elements of a brief lifestyle counseling approach.

DOI: 10.1201/9781003099116-7

6.2   GETTING STARTED

6.2.1   ASSESSMENT

Assessment typically includes a patient's degree of obesity, their dietary pattern, amount of physical activity, emotional problems, including stress, anxiety, and depression, and their current motivation and reasons for wanting to change. The patient's degree of obesity will help the health care provider determine the most useful intervention. Behavioral change strategies are typically most helpful for patients with a body mass index (BMI) of 25–40. Patients whose BMI's exceed 40 may need more intensive interventions, sometimes involving bariatric surgery [1]. Registered dietitians are the best professionals for assessing dietary patterns. If none is available, there are several assessment tools available such as the Healthy Habits and History Questionnaire, the Dietary Assessment Questionnaire, and others [2]. Physical activity can be assessed by asking patients the minutes per day they spend in brisk walking or similar activities. There are also questionnaires such as the 7-day Physical Activity Recall Questionnaire and others available [3]. Emotional problems frequently interfere with behavioral interventions. There are many questionnaires available for assessment, including the PHQ-9, the Beck Depression Inventory, and similar instruments [4–6]. They can be helpful in identifying patients, especially those severely depressed or suicidal, who will need referral to mental health professionals before beginning behavioral intervention.

Motivation to change is idiosyncratic. For patients who do not appear especially motivated to begin a behavioral change intervention, personalizing their risk factors, such as explaining how a 5% weight loss may lower their elevated blood pressure, plasma lipid levels, or plasma glucose levels, can sometimes be helpful in getting them started.

6.2.2   BEHAVIORAL MANAGEMENT STRATEGIES

Behavioral management strategies are aimed at helping patients develop for themselves the skills needed to achieve and maintain a healthier lifestyle. For patients with obesity, the goal of behavioral management is to help them adhere to a healthy diet and physical activity plan. Management involves dealing with cultural and environmental challenges, emotional factors, including stress, anxiety, depression, and other psychosocial issues. For health care providers, these toolbox strategies include setting goals, raising awareness, confronting barriers, restructuring beliefs, managing stress, preventing relapse, providing support, and writing contracts.

Setting goals. Patients oftentimes have unrealistic goals about losing weight [7]. Some will tell the health care provider that they want to lose 30% or more of their current weight, when most patients realistically will lose 5%–10%. At the beginning of intervention, it is important to encourage the patient to set relatively easy short-term goals such as increasing the number of minutes or steps of physical activity and then helping them focus on the psychological feeling of enhanced well-being that can oftentimes be quite motivating. Patients frequently feel good about achieving short-term goals and may be encouraged to try additional ones. It is important to reevaluate goals frequently and revise them as needed. These initial small changes may lead to some improvements in cardiovascular risk factors, and these benefits should be noted and applauded.

Raising awareness. Self-monitoring of behavior is important for achieving and maintaining a healthier lifestyle because it raises awareness of the behaviors needing to be changed [8,9]. For patients with obesity, it is critical to know what they are eating and how much they are exercising. Their awareness may not be enough for behavioral change, but it is necessary. Some form of food and exercise diary is important. The strategy involves three steps: self-observation, self-recording, and feedback. There are many ways to do this, such as simply asking the patient to write down what and how much they eat and how many minutes they exercise. The patient then looks up the calories of the food they ate and estimates how many calories they burned exercising, calculating about 5 calories per minute of walking, with 20 minutes equaling 100 calories. About 100 calories are burned for each 2,000 steps. Pedometers and other fancy devices can make it especially easy. Accuracy is not critical here, as most individuals underestimate their energy intake by about one third and overestimate their energy expenditure by about one half [10–12]. Remember, food and exercise diaries are critical not for their accuracy but because they help raise the patient's awareness of what they are eating and exercising. In our experience, we find that most patients do not like to keep diaries. Yet, if health care providers encourage their use, diaries will significantly increase a patient's chances of long-term success. One study reported that individuals who wrote the most words in their food diaries at the beginning of their intervention had lost the most weight 1 year later compared to fellow participants who initially wrote fewer words [13]. Diaries are an essential component of a behavioral toolbox. Additionally, to raise awareness of body weight, weighing on a regular schedule, such as once a day during the weight loss phase, and once a week during maintenance, is needed.

Confronting barriers. What barriers are preventing the patient from eating healthier and exercising regularly? Stimulus control strategies involve helping the patient identify and modify the barriers interfering with the person's lifestyle program [14]. Patients frequently struggle with their diet and exercise program because of environmental triggers or cues. The food and exercise diary, or a brief discussion with the patient, can help identify problems faced since the last appointment. Eating late in the evening, extensive travel, and eating regularly in restaurants are common barriers interfering with diet and exercise plans. Once identified, asking patients what they can do to solve these problems in the future can be helpful. Encouraging patients to come up with their own solutions to problems is usually better than the health care provider suggesting solutions for them. Planning sensible evening snacks ahead of time; carrying meal replacements or prepackaged, calorie-controlled meals when traveling; and calling restaurants ahead of time and asking for healthy meal suggestions are some potential strategies that can help manage these problems.

Restructuring beliefs. Oftentimes patients' beliefs, attitudes, thoughts, and negative feelings about themselves will determine whether a behavioral intervention will succeed or fail. Cognitive restructuring strategies help manage these factors by changing the way patients think about themselves [15]. For example, some patients with obesity appear to believe that losing weight will magically change their lives and that all their problems will disappear. Cognitive restructuring of beliefs is aimed at encouraging them to think about themselves in a more positive, realistic, and rational manner. Patients can learn to develop self-enhancing, self-affirming beliefs to help them stay focused. Having individuals come up with their own self-affirmations, repeated daily, is usually better than having the health care provider prescribe them. Watching professional football players and other sports professionals, we all know of stories about athletes who psych themselves up before the big game. It is the same principle here. Patients are asked to repeat to themselves their own personal affirmations five times a day. Repeating "just do it" or something similar can frequently serve as a motivator to encourage them in their behavioral change program. Having patients come up with simple affirmations such as "I will walk for 30 minutes today" can help serve as an impetus for lasting change. Writing their self-affirmations on a small card and reading them daily may also remind them to just do it.

Managing stress. Living through this current Covid-19 pandemic, we are all familiar with the role stress, tension, anxiety, depression, anger, boredom, loneliness, and other negative affective states can interfere with our otherwise healthy lifestyles, despite our best intentions. Stress is an especially damaging emotion and frequently contributes to over-eating and under-exercising [16]. For patients with obesity, once its sources are identified, there are several behavioral strategies that can help manage it and other negative emotional states when they are significantly interfering with the progress of the intervention [17,18]. Physical activity is an especially useful strategy for managing stress, in part because it helps raise the feeling of psychological well-being. Daily meditation is another one. Progressive muscle relaxation, a strategy involving tensing and relaxing muscles, can be easily learned and may lead to significant stress reduction.

Preventing relapse. Problem solving is important for the achievement of patients' goals [19,20]. Once reasonable, realistic goals have been agreed upon, problem solving helps identify potential barriers that may hinder the achievement of these goals. Brainstorming potential solutions to overcome these obstacles can be helpful. They may also increase patients' confidence in achieving goals and build self-efficacy to effectively face potential future problems. For example, we all stray from time to time. Health care providers can help patients understand that to err is human and that lapses are normal, expected, and manageable. They can encourage patients to anticipate situations where lapses may occur, such as during holidays, vacations, and visits to Las Vegas, and to develop behavioral strategies to cope with the challenges. The goal is not to prevent all lapses but to help patients better understand when they may occur and to prevent them from becoming relapses and total collapses.

Providing support. Strong support from family members, close friends, neighbors, colleagues at work, physicians, registered dietitians, counselors, and other health care providers can be powerful for patients trying to lose or maintain lost weight or make other healthy lifestyle changes [21]. Families that eat and exercise together can be wonderful support systems. Friends who exercise together can serve as motivators to each other. Support systems are oftentimes successful because they provide good role models, encourage each other in overcoming barriers and challenges, and allow for self-acceptance. Being part of a support group, patients may learn that if others can make positive lifestyle changes so can they. Unfortunately, sometimes supposed support individuals, such as a spouse or other family member, relative, or friend, may, for reasons of their own, try to sabotage the change process. Choosing the right support persons oftentimes makes the difference between success or failure.

Writing contracts. Behavioral contracts typically involve patients agreeing to make one or two healthy changes in their lifestyle and to carry them out between appointments with the health care provider [22]. The process involves signing a formal "contract" to that effect. Contracts are most helpful if the agreed-upon changes are short-term, realistic, and not too difficult, but a little challenging. An example might be a patient agreeing to increase the number of days or times per day walked. Another might be a patient agreeing to skip desserts at meals for 1 week or adding a new vegetable at the evening meal. The health care provider writes down the agreed to changes and both the patient and the provider sign the document making it "official." We have found that contracts will maintain motivation in the short term only and that new contracts with new behaviors need to be implemented at each session.

6.2.3 INCORPORATING BEHAVIORAL MANAGEMENT INTO INTERVENTION

When describing behavioral strategies separately, as we have in this chapter, it may appear that they are used independently. However, behavioral management strategies are almost always used as a "package," in combination with each other [23]. Few research interventions have tested any of these strategies as a sole intervention. The strategies are used together to improve adherence to a healthy diet and exercise. For example, raising self-awareness about caloric intake and physical activity behaviors is essential for weight loss and maintenance and should be used in conjunction with setting reasonable goals to encourage behavior change. Making gradual changes, such as slowly reducing calories and increasing physical activity, will encourage losing weight at a safe rate and relatively easy. Likewise, strong social support may help motivate these changes and, ultimately, long-term weight maintenance.

6.2.4 STREAMLINING BEHAVIORAL MANAGEMENT

Current guidelines for the behavioral management of patients with obesity recommend 60–90-minute weekly sessions, either individual or group, for the first 6 months, followed by biweekly, then monthly sessions [1]. A good group size is about 8 patients. The interventionist, who is typically a registered dietitian, psychologist, nurse, or other health care provider, should have received training in conducting behavioral counseling sessions. There are several advantages to either meeting with patients in groups or individually. The primary advantage of group sessions is that larger numbers of patients can receive intervention at the same time, and the group members can serve as role models and as a source of support to each other [24]. The primary disadvantage is that there is less time to tailor the behavioral strategies to each individual patient as the size of the group increases. Individual sessions of course provide more time for tailoring, but patients lack the support that groups may provide, and fewer patients can be seen by the interventionist. Overall, we prefer group sessions. In the perfect world, the behavioral strategies would be delivered by a multidisciplinary team of health care providers, including physicians, registered dietitians, exercise physiologists, and behavioral specialists. Other than well-supported research centers, it is not likely that many clinical sites are able to provide such a team. With limited time available, most health care professionals need to focus on the essential elements of a behavioral intervention. The most critical strategies for behavior change include: (a) raising awareness (self-monitoring), (b) overcoming barriers (stimulus control), (c) managing stress, and (d) providing support. The others, such as writing contracts, can be available in the interventionist's toolbox and used to a greater or lesser extent depending on the patient. A monthly 20 minute individual session involving a brief review of the food and exercise diary (or a discussion of the patient's diet and physical activity since the last session if the patient hasn't kept a diary), a review of goals from the previous session, a discussion of both old and new problems since the last session, and, finally, setting new goals for the next session, will get at most of the relevant behavioral issues.

6.2.5 BEHAVIORAL RESEARCH RESULTS

There are many excellent research studies and reviews documenting the efficacy of behavioral management strategies. In randomized, controlled obesity trials, the combination of strategies for increasing adherence to a healthy diet and exercise program delivered in weekly sessions over a 6-month period result in average weight losses of about 8% in patients with obesity [25]. This amount of weight loss will generally result in beneficial changes in blood pressure, blood lipids, blood glucose, insulin sensitivity, endothelial function, overall well-being, improved quality of life, and other factors [25].

Unfortunately, the long-term maintenance is not positive. Without continued intervention most individuals tend to regain some or all their lost weight over time. Few individuals will maintain all their losses for two or more years. Studies suggest that with extended intervention some patients maintain more modest but still clinically significant losses of about 5%. Remember to put this in perspective. Without any intervention, the average adult gains about 0.6 kg/year [26]. Although patients tend to gain weight after intervention, many do well, and the behavioral skills learned during intervention may benefit them when future obstacles and challenges occur [27].

6.2.6 LONG-TERM BEHAVIORAL MANAGEMENT RESULTS: THE GOLD STANDARDS

6.2.6.1 Diabetes Prevention Program

The Diabetes Prevention Program (DPP) is an outstanding example of an intervention for preventing or delaying the onset of type 2 diabetes in at-risk persons who are overweight/obese [28,29]. A total of 3,234 individuals at risk for type 2 diabetes were randomized to lifestyle modification intervention, metformin, or placebo. The goals of the study included a 7% weight loss and 150 minutes per week of physical activity. The lifestyle modification intervention consisted of an initial 16 sessions of diet, physical activity, and behavioral strategies, including those discussed earlier in this chapter. Participants initially were seen individually. After the first 24 weeks, the number of individual sessions was gradually decreased to usually monthly, and group sessions were added occasionally to help motivate and reinforce behavior change.

Results showed a mean weight loss at 1 year of 6.7 kg in the lifestyle modification group, compared with a 2.7 kg loss in the metformin group and 0.4 kg loss in the placebo group. At 4 years, the lifestyle modification group had a mean weight loss of 3.5 kg, compared with 1.3 kg in the metformin group, and 0.2 kg in the placebo group. Most importantly, the lifestyle modification group showed a 58% reduction in the incidence of type 2 diabetes compared to the placebo group, whereas the incidence in the metformin group was reduced by 32%. The lifestyle modification group was significantly more effective in reducing the incidence of type 2 diabetes than both the metformin and placebo groups. The Diabetes Prevention Program clearly documented the efficacy of a behavioral management intervention for significantly improving a healthy lifestyle. The American Diabetes Association also has recommended that patients with prediabetes be referred "to an intensive lifestyle behavior change program modeled on the Diabetes Prevention Program to achieve and maintain a weight loss 7% of initial body weight and increase moderate-intensity physical activity (such as brisk walking) to at least 150 min/week" [29]. The pioneering work of the Diabetes Prevention Program has since been expanded both in the United States and globally, including cultural adaptations in Finland, Australia, China, and India [30].

6.2.6.2   LOOK AHEAD

Look AHEAD is the largest, longest trial of the effects of behavioral management on the health of middle-aged individuals with type 2 diabetes and overweight/obesity [31–33]. It is a multicenter, randomized controlled trial to determine whether modest weight loss achieved through a healthy diet, physical activity, and behavioral management would reduce cardiovascular morbidity and mortality. A total of 5,145 adults with type 2 diabetes and overweight/obesity were randomly assigned to either an "Intensive Lifestyle Modification Intervention" (ILI) or to a "Diabetes Support and Education" (DSE) control group. The DSE group received three one-hour group meetings per year focusing on diet, physical activity, and support. Information was provided, but no behavioral strategies were taught.

The goals for the ILI group included a 7% weight loss and 175 minutes per week of physical activity, mostly walking. The ILI group attended 24 sessions during the initial 6 months. The number of sessions decreased in the second 6 months and in subsequent years. Participants were prescribed a daily goal of 1,200–1,800 calories depending on each individual's caloric needs. The ILI group was provided with liquid meal replacements as a form of portion control during the initial 6 months and were encouraged to replace two meals a day with a liquid shake (meal replacement) and one snack (a bar) and increase their intake of fruits and vegetables. During the second 6 months, shakes and snacks were reduced to a total of two per day. Individuals were encouraged to increase consumption of healthy low-energy-dense foods. Shakes and snacks were discontinued after year one. Participants were asked to walk at least 10,000 steps per day. Brisk walking, or similar physical activity, was prescribed at 125 minutes per week, which later increased to 175 minutes per week. The behavioral management consisted of the strategies described earlier in this chapter, including the use of the toolbox for individuals who struggled to meet the study's goals.

Results at the end of year one exceeded expectations, with the ILI group losing an average of 8.6% of their initial weight compared with 0.7% of the DSE control group. This significant loss was associated with a number of beneficial changes, including improved diabetes control and reduced cardiovascular risk factors in the ILI group compared to the DSE control group.

Results at the 9.6-year assessment showed the average weight loss for the ILI group was 6.0%, compared with 3.5% in the DSE control group. At every annual assessment, weight losses for the ILI group were significantly greater than the DSE control group. Although the trial did not meet its primary goal of significantly reduced cardiovascular morbidity and mortality, it has demonstrated the efficacy of behavioral management for long-term weight loss and maintenance. Look AHEAD has continued as an observational cohort study to assess additional long-term benefits of the initial behavioral intervention.

6.3   CONCLUSION

Behavioral management intervention is the key to the development and maintenance of a healthier lifestyle. Research demonstrates that behavioral management will remain the foundation for losing weight and adopting a healthier diet and exercise program for patients with obesity. The Look AHEAD trial, the largest and longest randomized intervention for patients with overweight/obesity and diabetes, has shown that through intensive behavioral management the elusive goal of long-term weight loss and maintenance is possible, along with significant improvements in cardiovascular risk factors and other benefits. Look AHEAD, along with other well-designed randomized controlled trials such as the Diabetes Prevention Program, documents that major benefits are attainable through well-tested behavioral management strategies. The challenge of health care providers is to incorporate the behavioral strategies utilized successfully in the Diabetes Prevention Program, Look AHEAD, and others and adapt them for use in their own clinical practices in primary care offices, hospitals, and other health care centers to help struggling patients better adhere to healthier lifestyles. Newer delivery systems, such as those that have significantly increased in use during this pandemic, including virtual sessions over the internet, apps, smartphones, and other mobile devices, may help extend interventions and contact with patients and improve long-term outcomes.

PRACTICAL APPLICATIONS

- Because no two patients are alike, clinicians can achieve better results with a "toolbox" of behavioral strategies to help tailor interventions to each patient's unique needs.
- Toolbox strategies include setting goals, raising awareness, confronting barriers, restructuring beliefs, managing stress, preventing relapse, providing support, and writing contracts.

- Behavioral management toolbox strategies are almost always used as a "package," not individually.
- Clinicians need to adapt behavioral management strategies for use in their own practices to help struggling patients better adhere to healthier lifestyles.

REFERENCES

1. Jensen M.D., Ryan D.H., Apovian C.M., Ard J.D., et al. 2013 AHA/ACC/TOS guideline for the management of overweight and obesity in adults: A report of the American College of Cardiology/American Heart Association Task Force on Practice Guidelines and The Obesity Society. *Journal of the American College of Cardiology*, 2014;63:2985–3023.
2. Thompson, F.E., Byers T. Dietary assessment resource manual (supplement). *Journal of Nutrition*, 1994, 124:2245S–2317S.
3. Blair S.N. How to assess exercise habits and physical fitness. In: Matarazzo J.D., Weiss S.M., Herd J.A., Miller N.E. Weiss S.M. (eds.) *Behavioral Health*. New York: John Wiley & Sons, Inc., 1984, pp. 424–447.
4. Beck A.T., Ward C.H., Mendelson M., et al. An inventory for measuring depression. *Archives of General Psychiatry*, 1961;4(6):561–571.
5. Steer R.A., Cavalieri T.A., Leonard D.M., Beck A.T. Use of the Beck Depression Inventory for Primary Care to screen for major depression disorders. *General Hospital Psychiatry* 199;21: 106–111.
6. Allison D.B., Baskin M.L. *Handbook of Assessment Methods for Eating Behaviors and Weight-Related Problems: Measures, Theory, and Research (Second edition)*. New York: Sage Publications, 2009.
7. Foster G.D., Wadden T.A., Vogt R.A., Brewer G. What is a reasonable weight loss? Patients' expectations and evaluations of obesity treatment. *Journal of Consulting and Clinical Psychology*, 1997;65:79–85.
8. Baker R.C., Kirschenbaum D.S. Self-monitoring may be necessary for success weight control. *Behavior Therapy*, 1993;24:377–394.
9. Wing R.R., Tate D.F., Gorin A.A., Raynor H.A., Fava J.L. A self-regulation program for maintenance of weight loss. *New England Journal of Medicine*, 2006;355(15):1563–1571.
10. Lichtman S.W., Pisarska K., Berman E.R., Pestone M., et al. Discrepancy between self-reported and actual caloric intake and exercise in obese subjects. *New England Journal of Medicine,* 1992;327(27):1893–1898.
11. De Vries J.H., Zock P., Mensink R.P., Katan M.B. Underestimation of energy intake by 3-d records compared with energy intake to maintain body weight in 269 nonobese adults. *American Journal of Clinical Nutrition*, 1994;60(6):855–860.
12. Tooze J.A., Subar A.F., Thompson F.E., Troiano R., Schatzkin A., Kipnis V. Psychosocial predictors of energy underreporting in a large doubly labeled water study. *American Journal of Clinical Nutrition*, 2004;79(5):795–804.
13. Tsai A.G., Fabricatore A.N., Wadden T.A., Higginbotham A.Z., et al. Readiness redefined: A behavioral task during screening predicted 1-year weight loss in the Look AHEAD study. *Obesity*, 2014;22(4):1016–1023.
14. McReynolds W.T., Paulsen B.K. Stimulus control as the behavioral basis of weight loss procedures. In: Williams B.J., Martin S., Foreyt J.P. (eds.) *Obesity: Behavioral Approaches to Dietary Management*. New York: Brunner/Mazel, 1976, pp. 43–64.
15. Foreyt J.P, Johnston C.A. Behavior modification and cognitive therapy. In: Mechanick J.I., Kushner R.F. (eds.) *Lifestyle Medicine: A Manual for Clinical Practice*. New York: Springer, 2016, pp. 129–134.

16. Ozier A.D., Kendrick O.W., Leeper J.D., Knol L.L., Perko M., Burnham J. Overweight and obesity are associated with emotion- and stress-related eating as measured by the eating and appraisal due to emotions and stress questionnaire. *Journal of the American Dietetic Association*, 2008;108(1):49–56.
17. Fabricatore A.N. Behavior therapy and cognitive-behavioral therapy of obesity: Is there a difference? *Journal of the American Dietetic Association*, 2007;107(1):92–99.
18. Berkel L.A., Poston W.S.C., Reeves R.S., Foreyt J.P. Behavioral interventions for obesity. *Journal of the American Dietetic Association*, 2005;105: S35–S43.
19. Marlatt G.A., Gordon J.R. *Relapse Prevention*. New York: Guilford Press, 1985.
20. Anton S.D., Foreyt J.P, Perri M.G. Preventing weight regain after weight loss. In: Bray G., Bouchard, C. (eds.) *Handbook of Obesity: Clinical Implications* (4th Edition). New York: Taylor & Francis, 2014.
21. Wing R.R., Jeffrey R.W. Benefits of recruiting participants with friends and increasing social support for weight loss and maintenance. *Journal of Consulting and Clinical Psychology,* 1999:67(1):132–138.
22. Foreyt J.P. Need for lifestyle intervention: How to begin. *American Journal of Cardiology*, 2005:96(4A):11E–14E.
23. Foreyt J.P., Pendleton V.R. Management of obesity. *Primary Care Reports*, 2000;6:19–30.
24. Renjilian D.A., Perri M.G., Nezu A.M., McKelvey W.F., Shermer R.L., Anton S.D. Individual versus group therapy for obesity: Effects of matching participants to their treatment preferences. *Journal of Consulting and Clinical Psychology*, 2001;69(4):717–721.
25. Johnston C.A., Moreno J.P., Foreyt J.P. Cardiovascular effects of intensive lifestyle intervention in type 2 diabetes. *Current Atherosclerosis Reports*, 2014;16(12):457–470.
26. Shah M., Hannan P.J., Jeffery R.W. Secular trend in body mass index in the adult population of three communities from the upper midwestern part of the USA: The Minnesota heart health program. *International Journal of Obesity*, 1991;15(8):499–503.
27. Kramer F.M., Jeffery R.W., Forster J.L., Snell M.K. Long-term follow-up of behavioral treatment for obesity: patterns of weight regain among men and women. *International Journal of Obesity,* 1989;13(20):123–136.
28. Knowler W.C., Barrett-Conner E., Fowler S.E., Hamman R.F. et al. Reduction in the incidence of type 2 diabetes with lifestyle intervention or metformin. *New England Journal of Medicine,* 2002;346(6):393–403.
29. American Diabetes Association, 3. Prevention or delay of type 2 diabetes: Standards of medical care in diabetes—2021. *Diabetes Care*, 2021;44(Supplement 1): S34–S39.
30. Johnston C.A., Absetz P., Mathews E., Daivadanam M., Oldenburg B., Foreyt J.P. Behavioral management of obesity: Enduring models, applications to diabetes prevention and management, and global dissemination. In: Fisher E.B., Cameron L.D., Christensen A.J., Ehlert U., Oldenburg B., Snoek F.J. (eds.) *Principles and Concepts of Behavioral Medicine: A Global Handbook*. New York: Springer Science+Business Media, 2018, pp. 835–860.
31. Wing R.R., Bolin P., Brancati F.L., Bray G.A., Clark J.M., et al., Cardiovascular effects of intensive lifestyle intervention in type 2 diabetes. *New England Journal of Medicine*, 2013;369(2):145–54.
32. Perri M.G. Effects of behavioral treatment on long-term weight loss: Lessons learned from the Look AHEAD trial. *Obesity*, 2014;22(1):3–4.
33. Lewis C.E., Bantle J.P., Bertoni A.G., Blackburn G. History of cardiovascular disease, intensive lifestyle Intervention, and cardiovascular outcomes in the Look AHEAD trial. *Obesity (Silver Spring)*. 2020;28(2):247–258.

7 Dietary Management of Overweight and Obesity

Nina Crowley, PhD, RDN, LD,
Medical University of South Carolina

Katherine R. Arlinghaus, PhD, RD
University of Minnesota

CONTENTS

7.1   INTRODUCTION

With a majority of American adults having overweight or obesity, weight management is one of today's greatest healthcare challenges. Rates of obesity and associated health conditions and healthcare costs continue to burden society. Obesity has been described as a chronic, relapsing disease process that is rarely, if ever, cured [1]. However, even modest weight loss of 5%–10% has been associated with significant improvements in cardiovascular risk factors [2]. Behavioral intervention is the cornerstone of obesity treatment and plays a role in all treatment plans, irrespective of the severity of obesity or treatment modality. Dietary modification is a key component of behavioral intervention for weight management. Specifically, appropriate dietary modification provides essential nutrients to achieve and maintain an optimal nutritional status while simultaneously producing an energy deficit to yield a reasonable weight loss or sufficient energy to prevent further weight gain, and balancing eating enjoyment with reductions in energy consumption to promote healthy

DOI: 10.1201/9781003099116-8

and sustainable eating patterns. This chapter will help guide clinicians through the dietary assessment, intervention, monitoring, and evaluation of patients with over-weight and obesity.

7.2 MEDICAL ASSESSMENT

Accurate assessment of weight status requires an office environment sensitive to the unique needs of patients with obesity. This includes having appropriately sized furniture, equipment, gowns, and scales that can weigh patients of all sizes. The assessment of overweight or obesity involves annual measurement of anthropomet-rics including height, weight, and calculation of body mass index (BMI; calculated as kg/m^2) to classify overweight and obesity using current classification methods. Weight and height are measured with the patient wearing light clothing or an exami-nation gown and no shoes. Patients identified as having overweight (BMI > 25 kg/m^2) or obesity (BMI > 30 kg/m^2) should be referred to a Registered Dietitian Nutritionist (RDN) for medical nutrition therapy (MNT) [3].

Measuring waist circumference in patients with BMI <35 kg/m^2 is recommended to provide additional information about other medical conditions associated with obesity, such as cardiovascular risk (>88 cm or >35 in for women; >102 cm or >40 in for men) [4]. A medical history and exam should query for cardiovascular risk factors like high blood pressure, hyperlipidemia, and hyperglycemia. The measurement of blood pressure, lipids, and glucose to assess for cardiovascular risk enables treatment to be matched to risk profile [4]. These markers are also critical to assess because they provide additional baseline measures from which patients' progress can be mon-itored and evaluated. This is important to help patients remain adherent to treatment plans during times of weight plateaus or when weight changes are not as expected.

During the medical examination and history, genetic syndromes as well as endo-crine disorders such as hypothyroidism, Cushing's disease, polycystic ovary syn-drome, and other metabolic conditions should be ruled out as contributing reasons for a patient's weight status. Acquiring medication history is also essential in identi-fying if any drugs are associated with weight gain and can be modified. For female patients, it is also important to inquire about the possibility of pregnancy before making weight loss recommendations. The Institute of Medicine has set guide-lines for total and rate of weight gain during pregnancy by prepregnancy BMI [5]. Recommendations for weight gain during pregnancy should be individualized based on prepregnancy BMI to improve pregnancy outcome, avoid excessive maternal postpartum weight retention, and reduce the risk of the child acquiring chronic dis-ease later in life [6].

7.3 NUTRITION ASSESSMENT

Medical nutrition therapy by the Registered Dietitian Nutritionist (RDN) will include a comprehensive nutrition assessment to obtain, verify, and interpret data needed to identify nutrition-related problems, their causes, and significance. It is an ongoing, nonlinear, and dynamic process that involves data collection and continual analysis of the patient's status compared to specified criteria [7]. The RDN should assess food- and nutrition-related history, anthropometric measurements, biochemical data, medical tests and procedures, nutrition-focused physical findings, and client history in order to individualize the comprehensive weight management treatment [8].

Assessment of food and nutrition-related history includes asking questions about beliefs and attitudes, including food preferences and motivations, food environment, access to fruits and vegetables, dietary behaviors, eating out, screen time, past dieting history, food allergies, medications, dietary supplements, and physical activity. Understanding the patient's weight history, family medical and health history, social history, living situation, and socioeconomic status are all factors to consider in a thorough assessment. Weight history includes questions about highest and lowest adult body weight, usual body weight (within the last 6 months), and, finally, the individuals' preferred body weight. Consideration of individual factors such as eating disorders, dieting history, pregnancy, and if a patient is receiving treatment for other health conditions that impact diet (e.g. chemotherapy, management of diabetes, renal disease) is a part of determining the appropriateness of a weight management plan.

Many RDNs are becoming proficient in performing nutrition-focused physical assessment, an examination of the body and physical function to help determine nutritional status, signs of malnutrition, and nutrient deficiencies [9]. A systems-based exam of regions of the body (i.e. skin, nails, hair/head, eyes, mouth, neck/chest) can help identify declining nutrition status and micronutrient deficiencies even when malnutrition is not present [9]. Assessment of body composition (fat mass and fat-free mass) can further help individualize the dietary intervention for weight loss. Because interventions aim to reduce fat mass while preserving fat-free mass, periodic assessment of body composition changes can help to measure changes during the intervention. Body composition testing can help provide additional, objective data, beyond weight/BMI to reinforce effectiveness and encourage patients to continue with their eating patterns.

7.4 DIETARY ASSESSMENT

7.4.1 DETERMINING ENERGY EXPENDITURE

Determining a patient's energy needs is a critical first step to creating a personalized dietary plan that creates the energy deficit needed for weight loss. Typically, an energy deficit of 500–750 kcal/day is recommended [3]. Energy needs can be determined by assessing total energy expenditure. An individual's total energy expenditure consists of three components: basal energy expenditure, thermic effect of food, and an adjustment factor for the physical activity level. The assessment of energy expended in the basal state is impractical. Resting energy expenditure, or resting metabolic rate, however, is practical to assess. Resting energy expenditure is considered to be ~10% above the basal state. This substitution works well in practice because the thermal effect of food, which is also difficult to measure, is approximately 10% of total energy expenditure. The overestimation of resting energy expenditure compared to basal energy expenditure can be substituted for the thermic effect of food. Therefore, determining energy expenditure requires assessment or estimation of both resting metabolic rate and energy expended through physical activity.

Resting metabolic rate should be measured through indirect calorimetry whenever possible [3]. Although reasonably priced, hand-held medical devices enable measurement of resting metabolic rate in the primary care setting; there are often times when measurement is not possible. The Mifflin-St. Jeor Equation (MSJE) is the most accurate predictive formula available for adults and has been found to predict resting metabolic rate within 10% of measured in most individuals [3,10,11]. Online and mobile applications utilizing the MSJE calculate energy needs particularly convenient and accessible. The simplified MSJE for males and females [11] is provided below:

$$\text{For females, REE} = 10 \times \text{weight}\,(\text{kg}) + 6.25 \times \text{height}\,(\text{cm}) - 5 \times \text{age}\,(y) - 161$$
$$\text{For males, REE} = 10 \times \text{weight}\,(\text{kg}) + 6.25 \times \text{height}\,(\text{cm}) - 5 \times \text{age}\,(y) + 5$$

To complete the estimation of total energy expenditure, physical activity level must be estimated. Assess the patient's current activity level and apply the appropriate activity factor of REE $\times$ 1.2 (sedentary), $\times$ 1.4 (low active to moderate), and $\times$ 1.6 (active). Subsequent adjustments for intentional activity or exercise (such as walking, biking, dancing, or exercise routines) are added as individuals engage in these activities and can be adjusted per day or averaged per week.

Given the depth of the physical activity and nutrition fields, separate examination of each of these areas is necessitated, and the specific role of physical activity in weight management will be discussed in more detail in other chapters. However, it is important to recognize that as the most modifiable components of energy balance, both physical activity and diet are inherent components of weight management that complement each other to create an energy deficit. In practice, the lines between physical activity and eating habits are more blurred and clinicians must assess both areas. The assessment of energy expenditure is a natural opportunity for the RDN to assess a patient's physical activity and sedentary behaviors. The assessment of activity patterns is crucial to being able to tailor recommendations. Although it is difficult to lose weight through increased physical activity alone, physical activity is a critical factor in the maintenance of weight loss [12]. As such, establishing regular physical activity routines is important at all weight management stages.

7.4.2 Determining Energy Intake

Once energy needs are determined, it is important to assess an individual's total energy intake and dietary composition. There are multiple ways to assess this including 24-hour recall, food frequency questionnaires, food records, and digital photography. Strengths and limitations of these methods are listed in Table 7.1.

TABLE 7.1
Dietary Intake Assessment Methods

Method	Strengths	Limitations
Food Record/Food Diary *Patients are asked to prospectively record intake for a specified period of time*	• Doesn't rely on patient memory • Can be completed in advance of dietetic visit • Portion sizes can be measured at the time of consumption • Data can be entered into dietary analysis program • Records of multiple days provide valid measure of usual intake for most nutrients	• Patient intake may change as a result of keeping a food record • Requires patient to be literate, numerate, and have portion size knowledge • High patient burden, time consuming • Relies on self-reported information
24-hours Recall *Patients are retrospectively asked about intake from the past 24 hours*	• Unlikely to modify behavior • Inexpensive • Low patient burden • No patient literacy requirement • Can be conducted in person or by telephone • Data can be entered into dietary analysis program	• Dependent on patient memory • Relies on self-reported information • Requires skilled interviewer • High inter-interviewer variability • Time consuming • Not representative of usual intake
Food Frequency Questionnaire *Patients complete a survey that retrospectively queries how often certain foods/beverages were consumed in a specified period of time*	• Low patient burden • Quick, inexpensive • Easily standardized • Useful screening tool	• Requires patient to be literate and numerate • Dependent on patient memory • Can be cognitively difficult for patient because food lists are not meal-based • Doesn't provide valid estimate of total intake or meal patterns
Diet History *Patients are interviewed about their usual eating habits*	• No patient literacy requirement • Low patient burden • Enables assessment of meal patterning, usual nutrient, and food group intake in one interview	• Dependent on patient memory • Requires skilled interviewer • Time consuming

Regardless of the method of dietary assessment, the goal is to determine a representative pattern from which dietary interventions and recommendations can be made. The establishment of such a pattern requires inquiry into not just what patients eat, but the time, place, and occasion of eating, as well as the method of preparation and portion size of foods eaten. These are important factors to determine sustainable changes. Mobile applications are now widely available for the assessment and self-monitoring of dietary intake. Patients may find tracking their intake more sustainable when using technology to assist in collection and monitoring.

7.4.3 DETERMINING EATING ENVIRONMENT AND READINESS FOR INTERVENTION

The practicalities of a patient's eating environment are important to assess. Recommendations are more relevant and feasible when the clinician understands the patient's access to food, food budget, delineation of responsibility for shopping and preparation, location of meals, cultural food practices, and with whom meals are eaten. Assessing the environment may help the clinician and the patient identify potential barriers to carrying out recommendations.

Although recommendations may focus on timing and meal frequency, there is limited evidence to support such recommendations [3]. Consistent with the principles of energy balance, solely changing the frequency of meals, without decreasing total energy intake, does not appear to induce a change in weight. For example, increased eating frequency has been associated with increased energy intake through snacks, and individuals rarely compensate at mealtimes for previously eaten snacks [13]. Lower calorie (<200 calories) snacks can help patients meet restricted energy intake goals. Breakfast consumption has not been found to lead to greater weight loss in randomized control trials [3]. However, research looking at the relationship between circadian rhythm and weight loss has indicated that eating a higher proportion of total energy intake earlier in the day may be helpful in weight loss [14]. Importantly, different timing strategies may be helpful for different individuals to adhere to reduced caloric intake. Assessing patients' schedules and lifestyle patterns can aid in the determination of how patients may be most successful in incorporating recommendations into their day.

Current guidelines also recommend assessment of motivation, readiness, and self-efficacy for weight management, based on behavior change theories and models (cognitive-behavioral therapy, transtheoretical model, and social cognitive theory/ social learning theory). Patient motivation is a key component of success in a weight loss program and is essential for any weight loss treatment. Motivational interviewing (MI) is a collaborative, goal-oriented method of communication between a practitioner and a client with a focus on drawing out a client's personal motives by allowing a person to find answers on his or her own. MI is believed to enhance motivation and self-efficacy, which are both considered to be key for making and sustaining behavior changes [8,11]. Asking a patient to rate on a scale from 0 to 10, the importance of behavior change and their confidence in being able to make the change is a quick and effective tool that all clinicians can use to gauge a patient's readiness to change.

7.5 DIETARY INTERVENTION

Before beginning intervention, it is critical for the registered dietitian to discuss expectations and set realistic weight loss goals together with the patient's input. As little as a 3%–5% weight loss has been shown to improve clinical cardiovascular markers, and 5%–10% weight loss improves even more cardiovascular risk factors [4]. While clinically meaningful, this amount of weight loss may differ from a patient's expectation. Addressing this potential mismatch prior to treatment can be important to a patient's success.

Many dietary approaches exist that facilitate the reduction of energy consumption. However, there is no one ideal dietary composition for weight loss or weight maintenance [3]. Low- and very-low-calorie diets focus specifically on the creation of an energy deficit. Very-low-calorie diets ($\leq$ 800 kcal/day) are only appropriate for use among patients with a BMI $\geq$ 30. While very-low-calorie diets have been shown to produce significantly greater weight loss than low-calorie (>800 kcal/day, usually 1,200–1,600 kcal/day) diets, short-term as well as long-term weight loss is equivalent between the two diets [3]. Meal replacements (liquids, bars, frozen entrees) are an effective strategy to increase adherence to the energy restriction imposed by either diet and are helpful with long-term weight management [3]. Meal replacements, which are generally formulated products such as shakes or portion-controlled entrees, have value because they provide a regulated amount of calories per serving, are usually fortified with essential nutrients and fiber, and are economical, safe, and convenient to use. They also provide a departure from normal eating patterns and can serve as a venue for reeducation about and/or reformulation of what foods can be substituted or reintroduced.

Other dietary approaches achieve a caloric deficit through the restriction of particular foods or macronutrients. Results of randomized control trials indicate no difference in the rate or magnitude of weight loss between diets of differing macronutrient composition when caloric intake is held constant [3]. On the individual level, however, it is likely that some approaches will be superior to others at helping a patient achieve the necessary caloric deficit and adhere to the diet long term. Additionally, cardio-metabolic outcomes may differ based on the dietary approach taken. For example, greater reductions in low-density lipoprotein cholesterol have been achieved through a low-fat diet compared to a low-carbohydrate diet; however, low-carbohydrate diets have produced a greater reduction in triglycerides and larger increase in high-density lipoprotein cholesterol than a low-fat diet of equivalent energy restriction [4]. In addition to weight loss, the Dietary Approaches to Stop Hypertension (DASH) diet with energy restriction produces reductions in blood pressure, and the Mediterranean diet with energy restriction may also result in cardiovascular risk factor improvements greater than those seen with low-fat diets [3].

Eating foods with low-energy density, the ratio of energy in a food to the weight of the food (kcal/g), may be a strategy for appetite control and subsequent achievement of energy restriction as it allows for a greater amount of food to be eaten relative to the energy consumed. It is important to note that for an energy deficit to occur using this strategy, high-energy-density foods must be replaced by low-energy-density foods [15]. Randomized control trials have shown that solely increasing fruits and vegetables (foods with low-energy density) does not produce weight loss [16]. Although the low-energy-density approach warrants further research, a lack of standardized methods and consensus on how to include beverages prohibits conclusions to be drawn on the efficacy of this strategy for weight loss at this time [17].

Similarly, because people typically do not compensate for energy consumed from beverages by reducing their energy from foods, it is recommended that caloric beverages be reduced or eliminated from the diet. For example, reducing sugar-sweetened beverage consumption has been shown in randomized control trials to aid in weight loss [18]. Nonnutritive sweeteners and fat substitutes have a role in the dietary management of overweight and obese individuals primarily because they can potentially lower caloric intake overall. For this reason, nonnutritive sweeteners have been endorsed by the Academy of Nutrition and Dietetics as a strategy to reduce energy intake by replacing sugar [19]. It is important that sugar and fat substitutes are used in the context of a regular diet, are used in moderation and balance with other foods, are appreciated for total energy and nutrient value, and do not replace other nutritious foods [19,20].

Finally, while total energy intake is of central importance, reductions in intake are too often accompanied by a decline in essential nutrients and overall quality of the diet. Dietary supplements should be considered when eating patterns are compromised, erratic, limited in choices, or <1,200 kcal/day [3]. Vitamin and mineral supplements should never be used in lieu of a healthy diet, and their use should be evaluated on a case-by-case basis.

Regardless of the dietary approach taken, close collaboration with the patient will help to create a realistic diet plan that takes into consideration weight loss and adequate nutrition. The dietary intervention should begin with the patient's usual pattern in mind. The diet plan should build on the strengths of the patient's current diet and incorporate modifications necessary to manage comorbid conditions. The usual food pattern derived from food records can be used to determine recommendations for change. Realistic strategies (e.g. increasing or decreasing food groups, assessing portion sizes, changing or substituting foods especially of high caloric and/or high fat value, and altering eating patterns when feasible) to impose a practical energy deficit should be decided upon through collaboration with the patient.

Although the concept of energy balance seems straightforward, great individual variation exists in weight loss treatment response and maintenance of weight loss. Dietary intake is complicated by the complex interplay between behavioral, psychological, and environmental factors. Individual variations in microbiome have been suggested to explain some of the individual variation in how much energy is absorbed from foods [21]. Established genetic and epigenetic variability underscore the importance of individualizing dietary intervention; however, it is unknown how to effectively do this [22]. Long-term adherence to dietary interventions is affected by how well the diet composition meets the most important of these established needs. The magnitude of weight loss achieved in the first few months of treatment is the best predictor of overall outcomes [23,24]. For these reasons, realistic goals and expectations for weight loss need to be addressed prior to beginning intervention, dietary approaches need to be decided on iteratively with the patient, and patient progress should be regularly monitored so that adjustments can be made as needed.

7.6   INTENSITY OF INTERVENTION

After dietary intervention and appropriate weight loss goals are determined with the patient, discussion about the intensity of the intervention is important. The AHA/ACC/TOS Guideline recommends referral for comprehensive lifestyle intervention for all patients encouraged to lose weight, including those for whom medical or surgical intervention is recommended [4]. Frequency of contact is an important characteristic in the achievement of weight loss. There is strong evidence for at least 14 medical nutrition therapy (MNT) encounters (group or individual) with an RDN over a period of at least 6 months [4]. High intensity, comprehensive weight loss interventions produce on average a weight loss approaching 5%–10% of initial weight [4]. Energy needs change as weight is lost. Continual monitoring and evaluation of energy requirements enable adjustments to energy intake recommendations to be made as needed. This will help to prevent the weight loss plateau that occurs around 6 months for many patients. For weight maintenance after weight loss, there is also strong evidence for monthly visits of MNT over at least 1 year [4]. Alternative modes of delivery, including electronically providing visits through phone, internet, or telehealth technology, may be indicated.

If patients are unable to meet health and weight loss goals, more intensive behavioral treatment, pharmacology, or evaluation for bariatric surgery should be considered as appropriate. It is important to note that dietary intervention plays an important role in all of these treatment approaches. Working with the patient's medical team, the RDN can tailor the dietary approach to be appropriate for the patient's specific treatment plan.

For those with a BMI ≥ 27 kg/m^2 and an obesity-related comorbid condition, or a BMI ≥ 30 kg/m^2, pharmacotherapy can be considered as adjunctive to comprehensive lifestyle intervention to achieve targeted weight loss and health goals [4]. Clinicians should be aware of the current FDA-approved medications indicated for weight loss through appetite suppression or absorption of fat. The potential risk of the medication should be weighed against the potential benefit of weight loss for the individual. Patients taking weight loss medications may be more likely to consistently adhere to a lower-calorie diet, increase physical activity, and experience weight loss and maintenance [4].

Patients who have a BMI ≥ 35 kg/m^2 with obesity-related comorbid conditions or BMI ≥ 40 kg/m^2 who are motivated to lose weight but for whom behavioral treatment has not resulted in sufficient weight loss should be offered a referral to an experienced bariatric surgeon with an interdisciplinary team of medical, nutritional, and psychological professionals for evaluation [4]. Several factors are involved in the decision to undergo surgery: patient motivation, treatment adherence, operative risk, optimization of comorbid conditions, and insurance coverage [4]. Although bariatric surgery is the most clinically and cost-effective treatment for severe obesity, less than 1% of patients with severe obesity undergo it. The decision to discuss surgical options is subjective and inconsistent, likely due to bias toward people with obesity and stigma associated with having surgery.

Patients rely on recommendations from primary care providers and other healthcare practitioners for treatment recommendations for chronic diseases, including obesity [25]. Providers often incorrectly assume that people with obesity are well-aware of their excess weight and report feeling ineffective at helping patients with obesity lose weight [25]. It is important for clinicians to be compassionate and recognize the complexities of the disease of obesity and following a shared decision-making approach. It is imperative that health care providers tell patients when their weight is a health concern, that there are treatment options for overweight and obesity, that the provider recommends treatment, and that the provider will support the patient throughout treatment and maintenance [4].

7.7   CONCLUSIONS

A number of dietary approaches have produced weight loss in the short term; however, long-term maintenance of weight loss remains a critical challenge. The patient's ability to adhere to a long-term diet is an important factor to consider when selecting the dietary intervention. Successful selection of the dietary approach taken in MNT depends on thorough assessment, monitoring, and evaluation of a patient's eating behaviors, environment, and level of readiness for intervention. Despite the critical role of dietary intervention in the treatment of obesity, reimbursement for MNT weight management varies by state and insurance provider. Future directions include continued progress in reimbursement for MNT for weight management by RDNs, consideration of "non-diet" approaches for people with obesity (e.g. intuitive eating), counseling to modify behavior, and greater focus on preventing weight regain after weight loss. It is critical that patients have a relationship with their health care team based on trust that the provider will continue to work with them, without judgment, even if they experience weight regain. Like other chronic conditions, management of obesity will be lifelong and will require a change in approach by provider and patient alike.

PRACTICAL APPLICATIONS

- Clinicians have a variety of tools available for nutrition assessment, most notably, referral to Registered Dietitian Nutritionists (RDNs) to provide medical nutrition therapy (MNT) for weight loss and maintenance.
- While nutrition assessment includes objective assessment of anthropometric data such as weight, waist circumference, and resting energy expenditure, clinicians should spend time discussing eating behaviors, environment, preferences, motivation, access, living situation, and history of disordered eating in order to individualize treatment recommendations.
- Dietary interventions generally reduce calorie intake through mechanisms designed to manipulate total calories, specific macronutrients, caloric density or texture of foods, or timing of eating occasions. Utilizing a shared decision-making approach will help create a realistic plan together with the patient that is both grounded in evidence and considerate of patient's preferences which can help with long-term adherence to the plan.
- It is important that providers appreciate their role as a trusted member of the patient's long-term care team and facilitate continual follow up and monitoring in order to recommend changes based on response, as well as to increase intensity to include pharmacology or surgical intervention when appropriate.

REFERENCES

1. Bray G.A. Obesity: The disease. *Journal of Medicinal Chemistry* 2006;49(14):4001–7.
2. Wing R.R., Lang W., Wadden T.A., Safford M., Knowler W.C., Bertoni A.G., et al. Benefits of modest weight loss in improving cardiovascular risk factors in overweight and obese individuals with type 2 diabetes. *Diabetes Care* 2011;34(7):1481–6.

3. Raynor H.A., Champagne C.M. Position of the Academy of Nutrition and Dietetics: Interventions for the treatment of overweight and obesity in adults. *Journal of the Academy of Nutrition and Dietetics* 2016;116(1):129–47.

4. Jensen M.D., Ryan D.H., Apovian C.M., Ard J.D., Comuzzie A.G., Donato K.A., et al. 2013 AHA/ACC/TOS guideline for the management of overweight and obesity in adults: a report of the American College of Cardiology/American Heart Association Task Force on Practice Guidelines and The Obesity Society. *Journal of the American College of Cardiology* 2014;63(25 Pt B):2985–3023.

5. American College of Obstetricians and Gynecologists. ACOG Committee opinion no. 548: Weight gain during pregnancy. *Obstetrics and Gynecology* 2013;121(1): 210–212.

6. Rasmussen K.M., Catalano P.M., Yaktine A.L. New guidelines for weight gain during pregnancy: What obstetrician/gynecologists should know. *Current Opinion in Obstetrics & Gynecology* 2009;21(6):521–526.

7. Academy of Nutrition and Dietetics. Nutrition Terminology Reference Manual (eNCPT): Dietetics Language for Nutrition Care. http://ncpt.webauthor.com. Accessed December 13, 2017.

8. Academy of Nutrition and Dietetics Evidence Analysis Library. Adult weight management: Executive summary of recommendations 2014. Academy of Nutrition and Dietetics. https://www.andeal.org/topic.cfm?menu=5276&cat=4690. Accessed December 13, 2017.

9. Esper D.H. Utilization of nutrition-focused physical assessment in identifying micronutrient deficiencies. *Nutrition in Clinical Practice* 2015;30(2):194–202.

10. Frankenfield D., Roth-Yousey L., Compher C. Comparison of predictive equations for resting metabolic rate in healthy nonobese and obese adults: A systematic review. *Journal of the American Dietetic Association* 2005;105(5):775–89.

11. Mifflin M.D., St Jeor S.T., Hill L.A., Scott B.J., Daugherty S.A., Koh Y. A new predictive equation for resting energy expenditure in healthy individuals. *The American Journal of Clinical Nutrition* 1990;51(2):241–7.

12. Donnelly J.E., Blair S.N., Jakicic J.M., Manore M.M., Rankin J.W., Smith B.K. American College of Sports Medicine Position Stand. Appropriate physical activity intervention strategies for weight loss and prevention of weight regain for adults. *Medicine and Science in Sports and Exercise* 2009;41(2):459–71.

13. Bes-Rastrollo M., Sanchez-Villegas A., Basterra-Gortari F.J., Nunez-Cordoba J.M., Toledo E., Serrano-Martinez M. Prospective study of self-reported usual snacking and weight gain in a Mediterranean cohort: The SUN project. *Clinical Nutrition* 2010;29(3):323–30.

14. St-Onge M.P., Ard J., Baskin M.L., Chiuve S.E., Johnson H.M., Kris-Etherton P., et al. Meal timing and frequency: Implications for cardiovascular disease prevention: A scientific statement from the American Heart Association. *Circulation* 2017;135(9):e96–e121.

15. Rolls B.J., Roe L.S., Meengs J.S. Portion size can be used strategically to increase vegetable consumption in adults. *The American Journal of Clinical Nutrition* 2010;91(4):913–22.

16. Kaiser K.A., Brown A.W., Bohan Brown M.M., Shikany J.M., Mattes R.D., Allison D.B. Increased fruit and vegetable intake has no discernible effect on weight loss: A systematic review and meta-analysis. *The American Journal of Clinical Nutrition* 2014;100(2):567–76.

17. Perez-Escamilla R., Obbagy J.E., Altman J.M., Essery E.V., McGrane M.M., Wong Y.P., et al. Dietary energy density and body weight in adults and children: A systematic review. *Journal of the Academy of Nutrition and Dietetics* 2012;112(5):671–84.

18. Tate D.F., Turner-McGrievy G., Lyons E., Stevens J., Erickson K., Polzien K., et al. Replacing caloric beverages with water or diet beverages for weight loss in adults: Main results of the Choose Healthy Options Consciously Everyday (CHOICE) randomized clinical trial. *The American Journal of Clinical Nutrition* 2012;95(3):555–63.

19. Fitch C., Keim K.S. Position of the Academy of Nutrition and Dietetics: Use of nutritive and nonnutritive sweeteners. *Journal of the Academy of Nutrition and Dietetics* 2012;112(5):739–58.
20. Position of the American Dietetic Association: Fat replacers. *Journal of the American Dietetic Association* 2005;105(2):266–75.
21. Krajmalnik-Brown R., Ilhan Z.E., Kang D.W., DiBaise J.K. Effects of gut microbes on nutrient absorption and energy regulation. *Nutrition in Clinical Practice* 2012;27(2):201–14.
22. MacLean P.S., Wing R.R., Davidson T., Epstein L., Goodpaster B., Hall K.D., et al. NIH working group report: Innovative research to improve maintenance of weight loss. *Obesity* 2015;23(1):7–15.
23. Unick J.L., Hogan P.E., Neiberg R.H., Cheskin L.J., Dutton G.R., Evans-Hudnall G., et al. Evaluation of early weight loss thresholds for identifying nonresponders to an intensive lifestyle intervention. *Obesity* 2014;22(7):1608–16.
24. Wing R.R., Hamman R.F., Bray G.A., Delahanty L., Edelstein S.L., Hill J.O., et al. Achieving weight and activity goals among diabetes prevention program lifestyle participants. *Obesity Research* 2004;12(9):1426–34.
25. Funk L.M., Jolles S., Fischer L.E., Voils C.I. Patient and referring practitioner characteristics associated with the likelihood of undergoing bariatric surgery: A systematic review. *JAMA Surgery* 2015;150(10):999–1005.

8 A Clinical Approach to Pharmacological Management of the Patient with Obesity

Magdalena Pasarica, MD, PhD
University of Central Florida

Nikhil V. Dhurandhar, PhD, FTOS
Texas Tech University

CONTENTS

DOI: 10.1201/9781003099116-9

8.1   INTRODUCTION

Weight loss is only one aspect of obesity management. A comprehensive obesity management should include strategies for prevention of obesity, weight loss and maintenance, and the management of contributors and consequences of obesity. The current obesity management guidelines highlight the role of pharmacotherapy in the management of people with excess adipose tissue (with a body mass index (BMI) at or above than 30 kg/m² or a BMI at or above 27kg/m² with at least one comorbidity) [1,2]. The recommendations state that weight loss drugs should be used as approved by the US Food and Drug Administration (FDA) in addition to lifestyle interventions, such as diet, physical activity changes, and behavior change counseling for inducing a negative energy balance, and to be followed by weight maintenance interventions with a health care provider (HCP) team.

However, at times HCP are reluctant to prescribe weight loss drugs for reasons of safety, probably due to widely publicized adverse effects of fenfluramine and dexfenfluramine experienced in 1997. These two drugs were linked with valvular heart defects and subsequently were taken off the market. How about the present times? Are the available next-generation weight loss drugs still the same? Currently, the FDA requires all weight loss drugs to be studied long-term for serious cardiac side effects in a large population before approval [3]. For example, a double-blind, placebo-controlled trial showed that in 12,000 patients with known cardiovascular disease or cardiovascular risk factors followed for 3 years, Lorcaserin (one of the drugs approved for long-term management of obesity) does not produce cardiovascular events more than placebo [4]. More than this, three of the five drugs approved for long-term management of weight loss include drugs approved and used safely for other indications for a long time without serious concerns for safety [5–7].

This chapter will discuss the FDA-approved pharmacological treatment of obesity with detailed clinical and practical considerations for HCPs who are considering pharmacological therapy in the management of patients with excess adipose tissue.

8.2   DRUGS APPROVED FOR PHARMACOLOGICAL MANAGEMENT OF OBESITY

Currently, there is one drug approved for short-term management of obesity and five drugs approved for long-term management of obesity. The indications, mechanisms, efficacy, side effects, black box warning, contraindications, formulations, titration schedule, and practical considerations for each of them are as follows.

8.2.1 Drug Approved for Short-Term Pharmacological Management of Obesity

8.2.1.1 Phentermine (Trade Name Adipex, Ionamin, Lomaira)

Indications: Phentermine is approved for short-term (a few weeks) weight loss as an adjunct to lifestyle changes in patients with the BMI of 30 kg/m^2 or greater or patients with the BMI of 27 kg/m^2 or greater in the presence of at least one weight-related comorbidity [8]. A chronic disease such as obesity requires chronic treatment. Therefore, it is hard to limit using a drug briefly for obesity management. Nonetheless, in practice, it is used for longer periods of time with acceptable side effects and efficacy [9].

Mechanism: It is a centrally active adrenergic drug, a sympathomimetic amine that stimulates norepinephrine release in synaptic terminals. With phentermine usage, patients can experience increased satiety and less hunger, craving, binging, and nighttime eating [8].

Efficacy: A meta-analysis of nine randomized controlled trials showed that patients treated with Phentermine (15–30 mg/day) and lifestyle changes for 2–24 weeks lost an additional 3.6 kg compared to the lifestyle change group only [10]. Another study used Phentermine with lifestyle changes for treatment of obesity for 156 weeks and showed a 6.1 kg additional weight loss compared to lifestyle changes only [11].

Side effects: The most common side effects of Phentermine include dry mouth, headache, insomnia, irritability, nervousness, euphoria, palpitations, tachycardia, and an elevated blood pressure. There have been a few case reports of primary pulmonary hypertension (HTN) and cardiac valvulopathy in patients taking phentermine [12]; however, these probably represent the background in the general population as it was not confirmed in controlled studies [10,11]. Drug abuse potential and addiction are reported as minimal [13]; however, it is still a DEA Scheduled IV drug.

Black box warning: None [8].

Contraindications: Phentermine is contraindicated in pediatric population, pregnant, and lactating patients; patients with uncontrolled HTN, arrhythmia, heart failure, hyperthyroidism, glaucoma, agitated states; history of stoke, coronary artery disease, drug abuse, reactions to sympathomimetic amines; and within 14 days of treatment with monoamine oxidase inhibitor (MAOI) [8].

Formulations: Phentermine is available as a 37.5 mg scored tablet, 15 and 30 mg capsule form, and 8 mg tablet [8,14,15]. The lower dosage formulation can be taken up to three times a day and is used for patients who are sensitive to a higher dosage. Therefore, it increases the options for a personalized treatment plan.

Titration schedule: Dosing should be individualized to obtain an adequate response with the lowest effective dose. Patients should avoid taking Phentermine before going to sleep to avoid sleep disturbance [8].

Monitoring: Patients should be monitored for changes in heart rate and blood pressure [8].

Practical considerations: The FDA approved Phentermine for short-term treatment of obesity in 1959, and it is now the most commonly prescribed obesity drug in the United States [16]. The popularity of phentermine over the other drugs is most likely due to the long-term data [17–19], the association with a rapid onset of appetite control, and improvement in patient attitude [17–19]. This is also the only drug approved for weight loss that can be found as formulary and at a relatively low price.

8.2.2 Drugs Approved for Long-Term Pharmacological Management of Obesity

8.2.2.1 Phentermine-Topiramate ER (Trade Name Qsymia)

Indications: Phentermine-Topiramate was approved as an adjunct to lifestyle changes in adults with a BMI at or above 30 kg/m^2 or at or above 27 kg/m^2 in the presence of at least one weight-related comorbidity [7].

Mechanism: Phentermine-Topiramate is a combination of the appetite suppressant phentermine together with the anticonvulsant Topiramate which acts on Gamma-aminobutyric acid (GABA) receptors to decrease appetite and increase satiety [7].

Efficacy: A 56-week phase 3 study of Phentermine-Topiramate was conducted in 2,487 adults who had overweight or obesity with two or more of the following comorbidities; HTN, dyslipidemia, type 2 diabetes, prediabetes, or abdominal obesity [20]. The drug doses were once-daily Phentermine 7.5 mg plus Topiramate 46.0 mg, or Phentermine 15.0 mg plus Topiramate 92.0 mg. All subjects received counseling for lifestyle management. The change in body weight was minimal in the placebo group (−1.4 kg) but was significant and dose dependent in the drug groups (−8.1 kg and −10.2 kg, respectively) [20]. Selected subjects (676) completed an additional 52 weeks of either active drug (Phentermine/Topiramate 7.5/46 mg, 15/93 mg) or placebo, in addition to lifestyle therapy. This length of treatment was not only well tolerated but caused more weight loss, clinically significant improvement in systolic and diastolic blood pressure, triglycerides, HDL cholesterol, LDL cholesterol, and insulin sensitivity compared to placebo. Interestingly, the incidence rate of diabetes significantly decreased in the Phentermine-Topiramate 15/93 mg group [1].

Side effects: At the higher dose, Phentermine-Topiramate causes dry mouth and paresthesia, constipation, insomnia, dizziness and dysgeusia, anxiety-related adverse events, and depression-related adverse events [20]. Due to the Phentermine component, rare serious adverse reaction include cardiac ischemia, tachycardia, pulmonary HTN and psychosis (see the Phentermine section for more information), and potential for abuse and dependence [7].

Black box warning: None [7].

Contraindications: Phentermine-Topiramate should not be used in pediatric patients, pregnant, and lactating patients; patients with uncontrolled HTN, arrhythmia, heart failure, hyperthyroidism, glaucoma, agitated states; history of stoke, coronary artery disease, drug abuse, reactions to sympathomimetic amines; and within 14 days of treatment with monoamine oxidase inhibitor. Caution for use in women of childbearing age [7].

Formulations: The trade name is Qsymia and is dispensed in 3.75 mg/23 mg, 7.5 mg/46 mg, 11.25 mg/69 mg, 15 mg/92 mg of Phentermine and Topiramate ER combination, respectively. The two largest dosages are contraindicated in patients with moderate or severe renal or hepatic impairment [7].

Titration schedule: Phentermine-Topiramate is to be taken once a day in the morning. HCPs are instructed to start with the lowest dose and increase to the next dose in 14 days. Due to the Topiramate component, medication should not be discontinued abruptly to avoid seizures, which occur in patients with predisposition to seizures [7].

Monitoring: Discontinue if, after 12 weeks, the weight loss is less than 3% with 7.5 mg/46 mg dosage or less than 5% with 15 mg/92 mg. Due to the Phentermine component, patients should be monitored for changes in heart rate and blood pressure. Because Topiramate increases the risk for cleft palate in pregnant women in the first trimester, there is a required negative pregnancy test before the beginning of the treatment and every 4 weeks after that. Patients should avoid concomitant use of alcohol and monitor irregular bleeding in women using oral contraceptives and potassium in patients using non-potassium sparing diuretics [7].

Practical considerations: Phentermine-Topiramate ER combination was approved in 2012; however, both drugs have been FDA approved and used individually for more than 20 years: Phentermine for short-term weight loss and Topiramate for seizures and migraines.

8.2.2.2 Naltrexone-Bupropion ER (Trade Name Contrave)

Indications: Naltrexone-Bupropion is indicated as an adjunct to lifestyle changes in adults with a BMI at or above 30 kg/m² or at or above 27 kg/m² in the presence of at least one weight-related comorbidity [21].

Mechanism: Bupropion is a dopamine and norepinephrine reuptake inhibitor approved for depression and smoking cessation that acts on the reward pathways. Naltrexone is an opioid receptor antagonist approved for alcohol and opioid dependence, which in this combination antagonizes the feedback loop that limits the anorectic effects of bupropion. Therefore, the combination works synergistically to suppress appetite and decrease food cravings [21].

Efficacy: The efficacy of this drug was studied in a 56-week double-blind, placebo-controlled study in 1,496 subjects with obesity or overweight (BMI at or above 27 kg/m²) with at least one weight-related comorbidity. The combination Naltrexone 32 mg/day and Bupropion 360 mg/day caused a significant weight loss of 6.4% vs 1.2% in the placebo-controlled group. Additionally, the combination drug caused an improvement in several cardiometabolic risk factors and increased control of eating impulses [22].

The drug was also studied in 505 subjects with overweight/obese and type 2 diabetes in a double-blinded, placebo-controlled trial. Naltrexone

32 mg-Bupropion 360 mg once daily for 56 weeks caused 5% weight loss compared to 1.8% in placebo group, and 44.5% of subjects achieved more than 5% weight loss compared with 18.9% in placebo. Interestingly, the drug also achieved a significantly greater reduction in HbA1C (−0.6%) compared to placebo (−0.1%). The percentage of subjects achieving the American Diabetes Association recommended target of 7% HbA1C was doubled in the treatment group compared to placebo (44.1% vs. 26.3%). Moreover, the treatment group observed an improvement in cardiovascular risk factors, triglycerides, and HDL cholesterol [23].

Side effects: Common side effects include nausea, vomiting, constipation, headache, dizziness, and insomnia. Serious adverse reactions include neuropsychiatric disorders, homicidal ideation, suicidality, depression exacerbation, HTN, hepatotoxicity, and closed-angle glaucoma [21].

Black box warning: Naltrexone-Bupropion ER has a black box warning the use in patients with major depression disorders or other psychiatric disorders as it may cause suicidality [21]. However, we note that three large studies showed that there was no increase in depression or suicidal events compared with placebo [22–24].

Contraindications: Naltrexone-Bupropion is contraindicated in patients with uncontrolled HTN, seizure disorders, anorexia nervosa, bulimia, and chronic opioid use; patients taking bupropion containing products, MAOI (during or within 14 days of discontinuation); and patients undergoing abrupt discontinuation of alcohol, benzodiazepine, barbiturates, and antiepileptic drugs [21].

Formulations: The trade name is Contrave and is dispensed in 8 mg naltrexone HCl/ 90 mg bupropion HCl extended-release tablets [21]. The maximum dose is 32 mg naltrexone HCl and 360 mg bupropion HCl for the general population; however, patients with renal and hepatic impairment need dose adjustment.

Titration schedule: Naltrexone-Bupropion is to be taken as 2 tablets twice a day by mouth. Patients should be started with 1 tablet in the morning for 1 week, then 1 tablet twice a day for 1 week, then 2 tablets in the morning and 1 tablet in the evening for 1 week, followed by 2 tablets twice a day as the maximum dose from then on as tolerated [21].

Monitoring: Patients with HTN should be monitored for changes in blood pressure and heart rate. If the patient has not lost at least 5% of initial body weight in 12 weeks, then the drug should be discontinued and an alternative management of obesity should be investigated [21].

Practical considerations: Naltrexone-Bupropion was FDA approved for long-term management of obesity in 2014. However, both component drugs have been approved by the FDA for almost 25 years, which speaks to the safety of this combination drug.

8.2.2.3 Liraglutide (Trade Name Saxenda)

Indications: Liraglutide is indicated as an adjunct to lifestyle changes in adults with a BMI at or above 30 kg/m^2 or at or above 27 kg/m^2 in the presence of at least one weight-related comorbidity [5].

Mechanism: Liraglutide is Glucagon-like peptide-1 (GLP-1) receptor agonist, which delays gastric emptying, increases satiety, and decreases appetite [5].

Efficacy: The weight loss effect of Liraglutide 3 mg/day was studied in a double-blind, placebo-controlled trial of 3,731 subjects with a BMI at or above 30 kg/m^2 or at or above 27 kg/m^2 in the presence of hyperlipidemia or HTN with lifestyle change counseling. After 56 weeks of treatment, Liraglutide caused 5.6 kg body weight loss more than the placebo control. In addition, Liraglutide treatment was accompanied by an improvement in the cardiometabolic profile [25].

Liraglutide has additional benefits in patients with prediabetes or type 2 diabetes and obesity. A large double-blind, placebo-controlled trial in 2,254 subjects with prediabetes and a BMI at or above 30 kg/m^2, at or above 27 kg/m^2 in the presence of comorbidities was undertaken for 3 years. A lower proportion of conversion to type 2 diabetes was observed in the Liraglutide group (2%) compared to the control group (6%), with a Hazard Ratio being calculated at 0.21 (95% CI 0.13–0.34). In addition, the subjects with prediabetes treated with Liraglutide lost significantly more weight compared to placebo (4.3% difference) [26]. In 1,361 subjects with type 2 diabetes with overweight or obesity, Liraglutide for 56 weeks caused 6% weight loss for the 3 mg/day dosage and 4.7% weight loss for the 1.8 mg/day dosage, compared to 2% weight loss in the placebo group [27].

Liraglutide also has benefits for patients with obstructive sleep apnea, as shown by a study where apnea-hypopnea index improved after 32-week study of treatment (−12.2 vs −6.1 events h (−1)), and this improvement was related to the degree of weight loss. This study also demonstrated that Liraglutide produced a significant larger percentage of weight loss compared to placebo (4.3% difference) and an improvement in HbA1C and systolic blood pressure [28].

Side effects: Common side effects include nausea, diarrhea, constipation, vomiting, headache, dyspepsia, fatigue, dizziness, abdominal pain, flatulence, and insomnia. Serious adverse reaction include thyroid C-cell tumor, medullary thyroid carcinoma, papillary thyroid carcinoma, colorectal malignancy, first-degree atrial ventricular block, and pancreatitis [5].

It is important to note that a large double-blind trial studied the cardiovascular side effects of Liraglutide in 9,340 subjects with type 2 diabetes and with high cardiovascular risk followed for 3.8 years. Death from cardiovascular cause, nonfatal myocardial infarction, or nonfatal stroke occurred in significantly fewer subjects treated with Liraglutide (13.0%) compared to placebo (14.9%) with a hazard ratio of 0.87 (95% confidence interval [CI], 0.78–0.97). The rate of death from cardiovascular events was lower in the Liraglutide (4.7%) compared to placebo group (6%). There was no significant difference in the rate of nonfatal stroke, myocardial infarction, and pancreatitis in the Liraglutide compared to the placebo group [29].

Black box warning: Liraglutide has a black box warning for use in patients with medullary thyroid carcinoma history or family history, or in patients with multiple endocrine neoplasia syndrome type 2 (MEN2) [5].

Contraindications: Liraglutide is contraindicated in patients with personal or family history of medullary thyroid carcinoma or MEN2, hypersensitivity to Liraglutide or pregnancy, and should not be used concomitantly with insulin or other GLP-1 receptor agonist [5].

Formulations: The trade name is Saxenda and is a prefilled injection pen with multiple doses of 0.6 mg increments. One pen has 3 ml solution which contains 6 mg/ml of active drug. Liraglutide is to be administered subcutaneously (abdomen, thigh, or upper arm) daily at any time of day, regardless of meal timing. Liraglutide should be used with caution in patients with renal or hepatic impairment [5].

Titration schedule: HCPs are instructed to start with 0.6 mg/day for 1 week, then increase the dose weekly to 1.2 mg, then 1.8 mg, then 2.4 mg until the maximum dose of 3 mg/day is reached [5].

Monitoring: It is recommended to monitor blood glucose in patients with diabetes, in order to avoid hypoglycemia. If after 16 weeks of treatment patient has not lost at least 4% of initial body weight, it is recommended to discontinue the drug and consider alternative treatment options for obesity [5].

Practical considerations: Liraglutide was approved by the FDA in 2014 for long-term weight loss; however, a different dosage (lower) of Liraglutide has been used as Victoza since 2010 for the treatment of type 2 diabetes.

8.2.2.4   Lorcaserin (Trade Name Belviq™, Belviq XR™)

Indications: Lorcaserin was approved by the FDA as an adjunct to lifestyle changes for chronic weight management in patients with a BMI of 30 kg/m^2 or greater or patients with a BMI of 27 kg/m^2 or greater in the presence of at least one weight-related comorbidity [6].

Mechanism: Lorcaserin is a selective serotonin receptor agonist on pro-opiomelanocortin neurons located in the hypothalamus that decreases food consumption and promotes satiety [6].

Efficacy: A 12-week study using different doses of Lorcaserin vs. placebo (in addition to lifestyle intervention) in 469 adults showed that there was more weight loss in the Lorcaserin groups proportionate to the drug dose [30]. Similar results were obtained in a 1-year Lorcaserin study performed in 4,008 adults with obesity and overweight [31].

Another 2-year clinical trial looked at the maintenance of weight loss and involved 3,182 adults diagnosed with overweight or obesity, who received placebo or Lorcaserin 10 mg twice a day plus lifestyle intervention. The treatment group showed significant weight loss at 1 year and maintenance of weight loss at 2 years. First year weight loss in the Lorcaserin treated group averaged 5.8 kg compared to 2.2 kg in the placebo group. Weight loss was maintained in year two in almost 70% of the Lorcaserin group compared to 50% for those on placebo [32].

Side effects: Common side effects include headache, dizziness, fatigue, nausea, dry mouth, constipation, and back pain. Serious side effects include valvular heart disease, serotonin syndrome, pulmonary HTN risk, bradycardia, anemia, priapism, depression, suicidality, abuse, and dependence [6]. We note that there were no increased cardiac valvulopathy findings in several studies of 52 weeks treatment compared to placebo [31–33]. Moreover, a multicenter, randomized, double-blind, placebo-controlled, parallel group study (CAMELLIA-TIMI) examined the incidence of major adverse cardiovascular events in 12,000 subjects with cardiovascular disease or multiple cardiovascular factors and found no difference in cardiovascular events of patients treated with Lorcaserin for 1 year compared to placebo [4].

Black box warning: None [6].

Contraindications: Due to the possible side effect of serotonin syndrome, it is recommended that Lorcaserin should not be used in conjunction with selective serotonin reuptake inhibitors, serotonin-norepinephrine reuptake inhibitors, monoamine oxidase inhibitors, triptans, bupropion, dextromethorphan, and St. John's wort [6].

Formulations: Lorcaserin is available as 10 mg tablets as trade name Belviq [6].

Titration schedule: Lorcaserin 10 mg should be taken twice daily or 20 mg XR to be taken once daily [6].

Monitoring: Lorcaserin should be discontinued if the patient does not lose more than 5% of initial body weight after 12 weeks of treatment. Patients should be monitored for symptoms of valvular heart disease, cognitive impairment, psychiatric symptoms, and priapism. If patients have diabetes, their blood glucose should be monitored to avoid hypoglycemia events [6].

Practical considerations: Lorcaserin was approved in 2012 by FDA for long-term weight loss. It is a modified form of Fenfluramine, an old weight loss drug that was taken off the market for causing cardiac valvulopathy.

8.2.2.5 Orlistat (Trade Name XenicalTM, AlliTM)

Indications: Orlistat is indicated for the management of obesity in conjunction with a reduced calorie diet [34].

Mechanism: Orlistat acts through inactivating gastrointestinal lipase thereby partially inhibiting the digestion of ingested fat. This action results in a decrease in fat absorption and energy intake, and the promotion of malabsorption [34].

Efficacy: In a 2-year study, subjects treated with Orlistat (120 mg three times a day) lost nearly 10% body weight in the first year compared to 5% weight loss in the placebo group, and fasting low-density lipoprotein cholesterol and insulin levels improved [35]. Other studies showed improvement in glucose metabolism and a reduction in high blood pressure [36,37].

Side effects: Common side effects include oil-spotting, flatus with discharge, fecal urgency, and fecal incontinence. Considering that the drug reduces fat digestion, these side effects are more if the diet contains higher fat. Serious adverse effects of Orlistat include hypersensitivity, anaphylaxis, angioedema, leukocytoclastic vasculitis, fat-soluble vitamin deficiency, hepatotoxicity, nephrotoxicity, and oxalate nephropathy [34].

Black box warning: None [34].

Contraindications: Patients with chronic malabsorption syndrome and cholestasis should not take Orlistat [34].

Formulations: The trade name Xenical contains 120 mg active substance to be taken 3 times a day. The trade name Alli is available over the counter and contains 60 mg of active drug to be taken three times a day, in conjunction with a reduced calorie and low-fat diet [34].

Titration schedule: none [34].

Monitoring: Monitor for side effects as indicated [34].

Practical considerations: FDA approved Orlistat for weight loss and weight maintenance in 1999 as Xenical and in 2007 approved Alli as an over-the-counter medicine. Several attempts to decrease the inconvenient gastrointestinal side effects caused by Orlistat have been made without any success [38].

8.3 A PRACTICAL APPROACH TO PHARMACOLOGICAL MANAGEMENT OF OBESITY: A TREATMENT ALGORITHM

Once it is determined the patient meets the indications for using weight loss drugs (see above), the management can be approached in a stepwise manner to maximize the rate of success.

8.3.1 STEP 1. PRE-TREATMENT DISCUSSION

Before initiating the pharmacological management of obesity, there are certain facts that need to be clearly discussed with the patient to correct popular myths about obesity and weight loss drugs.

Fact 1: Obesity is not a character flaw, but a serious condition, and should be treated accordingly (https://media.npr.org/documents/2013/jun/ama-resolution-obesity.pdf). **Fact 2**: The FDA has approved five drugs for the management of obesity and just like any other FDA-approved drugs, weight loss drugs have potential risks. The risk-benefit ratio needs due consideration for obesity management, just like that for any other illness [5–7,21,34]. **Fact 3**: Weight loss drugs are approved to be used along with lifestyle changes for weight loss, and therefore are not substitutes but supplements to behavior change. Except for orlistat, they empower a person to adhere to the behavior changes implemented by decreasing appetite and craving and increasing satiety [5–7,21,34]. **Fact 4**: Since obesity is a chronic condition, weight loss drugs should be used long term for the management of obesity. Just like any other chronic disease, when drugs are discontinued, the disease may rebound, i.e. weight loss is regained [32]. **Fact 5**: Few patients treated with obesity reach their goal weight with or without drugs [39]. However, weight loss improves comorbidities [1,22,23,26–28] and quality of life [40]. The provider's goal should be to help patient achieve at least 5%–10% weight loss, which is sufficient to start health improvement. **Fact 6**: Patients have to be able and willing to comply with the medical regimen and lifestyle changes to improve the chances of success [41]. Therefore, a relevant motivation should be identified in discussion with the patient. It is important to note that improvement in health with weight loss is usually not a compelling motivator from a patient's standpoint and if used as the only argument by a provider, it may be unsuccessful. A more careful discussion to identify relevant goals may be needed. For example, being able to play sports with the family, or go dancing with friends without experiencing knee pain, or having improved sexual health could be some objectives that the patients may aspire to achieve.

8.3.2   Step 2. Drug Optimizations

HCPs should obtain a comprehensive history and perform a comprehensive physical exam of the patients treated for excess adipose tissue. In particular, the history should include the lifestyle history and weight gain/loss history with identifications of concomitant events for changes in weight. The physical should include signs and symptoms of obesity-related complications (e.g. complaints involving weight-bearing joints, edema, breathing, or lung-related conditions) or causes for weight gain (e.g. hypothyroidism, Cushing's disease).

If the history and/or physical suggest a secondary cause for obesity, then patients should be screened for those conditions and treated as needed. If any new obesity complications are diagnosed, then they need to be treated appropriately or referred to the appropriate medical HCPs.

The next step is to review the list of medications that a patient is taking and consider replacing any drugs promoting weight gain with drugs that are weight neutral or that promote weight loss. If the provider treating obesity is not the prescribing provider for some of the medication, then clear justified recommendations could be made to the prescribing provider with appropriate follow-up. For example, in patients with type 2 diabetes, HCPs should consider switching weight-promoting medicine like the thiazolidinedione class of drugs or sulfonylureas, with a weight-losing anti-diabetes drug (metformin, pramlintide, liraglutide). For the treatment of hypertension (HTN), it may be worth considering either angiotensin-converting enzyme inhibitor, angiotensin receptor blocker, or calcium channel blocker, to avoid beta-blockers, which have a weight gaining effect. For the treatment of depression, HCPs should consider switching mirtazapine or tricarboxylic acid drugs with drugs like bupropion that promote weight loss. For women interested in contraception, HCPs should consider methods other than weight gaining injectable or oral medicines. For patients with rheumatoid arthritis or other chronic inflammatory disease, it is recommended to consider nonsteroidal anti-inflammatory drugs or disease-modifying antirheumatic drugs instead of steroids. For seizures, HCPs should consider the use of topiramate and zonisamide instead of gabapentin or valproate to optimize weight loss [42,43].

8.3.3   Step 3. Rule-Out Pharmacotherapy Choices

Once the decision to use pharmacotherapy for weight loss has been made and patient has been medically optimized, HCPs need to identify the drug to initiate weight loss treatment. If the patient needs only a short-term weight loss treatment, then phentermine may be a drug of choice.

If the patient needs long-term weight loss treatment, then the available drugs are Phentermine-Topiramate, Naltrexone-Bupropion, Lorcaserin, Liraglutide, and Orlistat. We recommend a systematic approach that starts with an initial step to ruling-out drug choices based on patient age, medical history, current pharmacological treatment, preference for medicine administration route, side effects, and medication cost.

If the patient is 12 years old or younger, there are no FDA drugs approved for long-term weight loss. If patient is between 12 and 18 years old, the only available choice is Orlistat. Patients 18 years old or older have all the 5 drugs available for long-term weight loss treatment [5–8,21,34].

For this step, history about pregnancy, lactation, and comorbidities is relevant. Even though only Phentermine-Topiramate is labeled as a teratogen, none of the other drugs is approved for pregnant or lactating women due to lack of safety data [5–8,21,34]. The main contraindications based on the systems affected include the following. If the patient has glaucoma or unstable cardiovascular disease, then Phentermine/Topiramate should not be used. If the patient has severe renal or liver impairment, or medullary thyroid carcinoma or MEN2, Liraglutide is contraindicated. Naltrexone-Bupropion is contraindicated for bulimia or anorexia [5–8,21,34].

The current pharmacological treatment is also important. The main drugs that rule out weight loss drugs are as follows. If patient is taking selective serotonin reuptake inhibitors (SSRIs), serotonin-norepinephrine reuptake inhibitors, and/or Bupropion, then Lorcaserin is not indicated. If patient is taking monoamine oxidase inhibitor, Lorcaserin, Phentermine-Topiramate ER, and Naltrexone/Bupropion should be avoided. If patient takes opioids as a chronic treatment then Naltrexone-Bupropion is not indicated. If patient is taking warfarin, anti-epileptics, levothyroxine, or cyclosporine, Orlistat should be avoided in order to avoid modified absorption of active substance [5–8,21,34].

Patients' dislike for or inability to comply with a certain administration route and frequency is common and should be considered. Liraglutide is to be administered subcutaneously using a pen, which may not be accepted by some patients and therefore could be used to rule out drug choices. All the other drugs are administered orally. For these, the frequency of administration may consider an impediment for some patients and a reason to rule out some medication choices. Phentermine-Topiramate is administered once daily. Naltrexone-Bupropion and Lorcaserin are administered twice daily. Orlistat is administered three times a day [5–8,21,34].

Another important factor to rule out medication choices is the possible side effect profile. Patients should decide which potential risks they are willing to take. For women of childbearing age, congenital malformation may be caused by Phentermine-Topiramate if taken in the first trimester of pregnancy. Other examples of possible side effects are organized by systems in Table 8.1 [5–8,21,34].

Cost is also a very valid concern for patients, especially because most insurances do not yet cover weight loss drugs. The most inexpensive obesity drugs are Orlistat and Phentermine-Topiramate. Naltrexone-Bupropion price is mid-level, while the other drugs are reported as expensive [42].

8.3.4   STEP 4. RULE-IN PHARMACOTHERAPY CHOICES

The next step in choosing a weight loss medication is to rule in pharmacotherapy choices to provide additional advantages like concomitant improvement of other comorbidities, maximum effect on certain behaviors, and efficacy potential.

TABLE 8.1
Possible Side Effects of Weight Loss Drugs

Cardiovascular System

Increased heart rate	Liraglutide
	Naltrexone/Bupropion
	Phentermine/Topiramate
Decreased heart rate	Lorcaserin
Increased blood pressure	Naltrexone/Bupropion

Pulmonary System

Dry cough	Lorcaserin

Gastrointestinal System

Nausea	Liraglutide
	Lorcaserin
	Naltrexone/Bupropion
Constipation	Liraglutide
	Naltrexone/Bupropion
Pancreatitis	Liraglutide
Fecal urgency, oily stools	Orlistat
Cholelithiasis	Orlistat
Nephrolithiasis	Orlistat

Neurologic System

Dizziness	Naltrexone/Bupropion
	Phentermine/Topiramate
Headache	Naltrexone/Bupropion
	Lorcaserin
	Liraglutide
Insomnia	Naltrexone/Bupropion
	Phentermine/Topiramate
Inattention	Phentermine/Topiramate
	Lorcaserin
Seizures	Naltrexone/Bupropion
Paresthesia	Phentermine/Topiramate
Neuroleptic malignant sdr.	Lorcaserin
Metallic taste	Phentermine/Topiramate

Psychiatric System

Depression	Naltrexone/Bupropion
Serotonin sdr.	Lorcaserin

Patients' current comorbidities should be an important consideration when selecting a new drug. Weight loss by itself improves obesity-associated diseases, but as
seen in the previous sections, weight loss drugs may have additional benefits and,
therefore, can be used to improve conditions besides obesity. For example, if patient
has migraines, HCPs should consider the use of Phentermine-Topiramate. If patient
has type 2 diabetes or pre-diabetes, Liraglutide or Lorcaserin may be considered. If
quitting smoking is desired or the patient has mild depression, Naltrexone-Bupropion
may be beneficial.

If food craving is considered by the patient as the major contributor to excess
food intake, then Phentermine-Topiramate or Naltrexone-Bupropion may be considered. When a patient reports dissatisfaction with not feeling full when following a
calorie-restrictive diet, Liraglutide or Lorcaserin may be considered. All long-term
weight loss drugs (except Orlistat) help to have a lower appetite and in turn increase
compliance to a low-calorie diet [5–8,21, 4].

One of the most frequently asked questions from the patients is which medicine is most effective. This is different for each patient depending on what are the
causes for excess weight gain. Currently, we know that the average weight loss
caused by Phentermine-Topiramate is 7%–9%, 5%–6% by Liraglutide, 3%–5% by
Naltrexone-Bupropion, 3%–4% by Lorcaserin, and 2%–3% by Orlistat. This is the starting point for a discussion about effectiveness, with the note that each patient is different
and may have a weight loss response that is different than the "mean weight loss" noted.
Also, that drugs are supplements to lifestyle changes and not substitutes [5–8,21,34,44].

8.3.5   STEP 5. PRESCRIBE MEDICINE USING THE RECOMMENDED TITRATION SCHEDULE, WATCH OUT FOR SIDE EFFECTS AND MONITOR EFFICACY

When using Phentermine-Topiramate, Naltrexone-Bupropion, or Liraglutide for
management of obesity, HCPs should follow the recommended titration schedule as
mentioned in the previous section. Side effects (described in previous section) should
be carefully monitored, and if not tolerated or clinically relevant, medication should
either be discontinued or kept at lower dosages [5–8,21,34]. As with any other symptom or sign, a detailed history should confirm that the presented complaint is not due
to a different disease or drug.

The weight of the patient should be carefully monitored also, with a minimal target of 4%–5% weight loss in 12 weeks [5–8,21,34]. If this target is not achieved, then
a different drug for obesity management, or referral to bariatric surgery or optimiz-
ing the lifestyle change intervention may be needed. The change in behavior could be
hindered by multiple facts, including certain barriers, inappropriate goals, and aber-
rant eating behaviors. Some patients may need to attend a comprehensive behavior
weight loss program or very low-calorie diet program.

8.3.6   STEP 6. CONCOMITANT MANAGEMENT OF CHRONIC COMORBIDITIES

Monitoring the progression of the diseases improved by weight loss is needed. For
example, patients with type 2 diabetes undergoing a concomitant treatment with
drugs for weight loss should be advised to monitor their blood glucose more often

and report any change in glucose patterns to the provider. Patients with hypertension should also be instructed to monitor their blood pressure every morning at home and report any change in pattern. This will ensure the drug dose is adjusted to match the need. Patients with hyperlipidemia should be monitored with fasting blood lipids after 3 months of the program so that the management plan could be readjusted as needed.

If the provider prescribing weight loss drugs is the provider for treating other obesity comorbidities, then written recommendations for increased follow-up and possible need for management optimizations should be sent to the respective provider.

8.4   PRACTICE CONSIDERATIONS BEFORE PRESCRIBING DRUGS FOR WEIGHT LOSS

8.4.1   PREPARE YOUR HCPS FOR PRESCRIBING DRUGS FOR WEIGHT LOSS

It should be noted that three of the obesity drugs are DEA Schedule IV: Phentermine, Phentermine-Topiramate, and Lorcaserin. Therefore, HCPs should follow all the local guidelines for prescribing any drug that is schedule IV as defined by the DEA. One drug (Phentermine-Topiramate) has a risk evaluation and mitigation strategy in place, and therefore all prescribing HCPs and dispensing pharmacies need a special certification [7, 45] obtained from the Qsymia website. This is meant to prevent congenital effects, which can occur if Topiramate is taken in the first trimester of pregnancy. It is recommended that Qsymia can be prescribed to women of childbearing age only if they have either (a) an intrauterine device; or (b) tubal ligation/hormonal contraception and use a barrier method; or (c) use two barrier methods. HCPs can also seek out comprehensive education in obesity medicine by conducting training and obtaining a certification from the American Board of Obesity Medicine (www.abom.org). However, this certification is not required for managing obesity with drugs for weight loss.

8.4.2   PREPARING FOR INTRODUCING PHARMACOLOGICAL MANAGEMENT OF OBESITY

All the drugs approved by the FDA for short-term or long-term weight loss should be used as indicated, in addition to counseling and education for lifestyle changes. And, as per recent obesity management guidelines [1,2], the lifestyle changes should match the characteristics of comprehensive intensive lifestyle intervention. This is an important aspect that needs to be considered by clinicians, practice managers, and owners of primary care practices. Offering the weight loss drugs, without lifestyle change interventions may not result in the desired/studied weight loss effects.

The clinic environment also needs attention. The furniture and medical equipment should be appropriate for the management of patients with excess weight. The staff needs to be trained in managing problems that are associated with excess weight.

Another fact that clinicians need to consider is that in some states there are a special set of laws associated with the prescription of obesity drugs. For example in Florida, HCPs who prescribe obesity drugs need to get a written informed consent from patients and post the weight-loss consumer bill of rights in the treatment room (http://www.leg.state.fl.us/statutes/index.cfm?App_mode=Display_Statute&URL =0500-0599/0501/Sections/0501.0575.html; https://www.flrules.org/gateway/ruleno. asp?id=64B8-9.012).

8.5   SUMMARY AND CONCLUSIONS

Obesity is a chronic disease that requires lifelong treatment. Currently, there is no cure for obesity. However, in the United States, six drugs with relatively good safety profile are approved for short- and long-term obesity management. Just like with any other drug, careful selection of a drug, its dose and duration, follow up and continuous assessment of efficacy, and due diligence on recognizing side effects are mandatory. In addition to the usual requirements for pharmacotherapy, HCPs need to be aware of extra state laws regarding weight loss management with pharmacotherapy.

As most patients want either to lose weight or maintain their weight, and obesity is associated with multiple comorbidities from various specialties, it seems that not only obesity medicine specialists, but primary care providers should be prepared to treat patients with obesity. In some cases, for which pharmacotherapy is indicated, they will need to prescribe, monitor, and optimize the treatment with weight loss drugs. A lot of progress has been made in this direction. First, obesity was declared a disease by the American Medical Association in 2013 (https://media. npr.org/documents/2013/jun/ama-resolution-obesity.pdf), which should increase the number of insurance companies covering obesity management with reimbursement of HCPs time and reasonable co-pays for patients. Second, an Obesity Medicine certification has been developed and is available for any provider to complete in order to become experts in the clinical management of obesity (http://abom.org/). Third, obesity medicine competencies have been developed, in order to target objectives for educational activities and ready-to-use peer-reviewed educational activities are published [46,47]. Obesity plays a substantial role in the development of other comorbidities such as diabetes, hypertension, cardiovascular disease, and cancer and many more. It is not enough to only focus on those comorbidities and leave obesity untreated. Similarly, effective treatment of obesity can dramatically improve many of the obesity-dependent comorbidities, which should be monitored as a part of obesity management.

Obesity is a complex and chronic disease and not a behavioral issue or moral failure. While negative energy balance is necessary for weight loss, it is extremely difficult for a patient to chronically eat less than what their body or mind is prompting to do. Pharmacological treatment of obesity is intended to empower individual's long-term adherence to a lower calorie diet.

Next-generation obesity medications have much better safety and efficacy profiles. However, caution is needed in carefully selecting appropriate patients and monitoring progress. As newer and better drugs are discovered and approved, they add to the choices available to a provider so that patient's need, health profile, and response could be matched more appropriately with drugs that would most benefit them with least side effects.

PRACTICAL APPLICATIONS

1. Follow the most updated guidelines for comprehensive obesity management.
2. Select an obesity drug by considering the patients' demographics, medical and social history, current medications, and personal preferences.
3. During the treatment of obesity, monitor for the control of the obesity-related diseases and adjust the treatment as needed.
4. If a response to an obesity drug is poor, or if it causes non-tolerable side effects, then the drug should be discontinued and an alternative approach should be discussed with the patient (including other drugs).

REFERENCES

1. Garvey, W.T., et al., American Association of Clinical Endocrinologists and American College of Endocrinology Comprehensive Clinical Practice Guidelines for Medical Care of Patients with Obesity. *Endocr Pract*, 2016. **22**(Suppl 3): pp. 1–203.
2. Jensen, M.D., et al., 2013 AHA/ACC/TOS guideline for the management of overweight and obesity in adults: A report of the American College of Cardiology/American Heart Association Task Force on Practice Guidelines and The Obesity Society. *Circulation*, 2014. **129**(25 Suppl 2): pp. S102–38.
3. Colman, E., Food and drug administration's obesity drug guidance document: A short history. *Circulation*, 2012. **125**(17): pp. 2156–64.
4. Bohula, E.A., et al., Cardiovascular safety of lorcaserin in overweight or obese patients. *N Engl J Med*, 2018. **379**(12): pp. 1107–1117.
5. Saxenda. Available from: https://www.novo-pi.com/saxenda.pdf.
6. Belviq. Available from: https://www.accessdata.fda.gov/drugsatfda_docs/label/2012/022529lbl.pdf.
7. Qsymia. Available from: https://www.qsymia.com/pdf/prescribing-information.pdf.
8. Adipex. Available from: https://www.accessdata.fda.gov/drugsatfda_docs/label/2012/085128s065lbl.pdf.
9. Hampp, C., E.M. Kang, and V. Borders-Hemphill, Use of prescription antiobesity drugs in the United States. *Pharmacotherapy*, 2013. **33**(12): pp. 1299–307.
10. Li, Z., et al., Meta-analysis: Pharmacologic treatment of obesity. *Ann Intern Med*, 2005. **142**(7): pp. 532–46.
11. Hendricks, E.J., et al., Blood pressure and heart rate effects, weight loss and maintenance during long-term phentermine pharmacotherapy for obesity. *Obesity (Silver Spring)*, 2011. **19**(12): pp. 2351–60.
12. Rich, S., et al., Anorexigens and pulmonary hypertension in the United States: Results from the surveillance of North American pulmonary hypertension. *Chest*, 2000. **117**(3): pp. 870–4.
13. Griffiths, R.R., J.V. Brady, and L.D. Bradford, Predicting the abuse liability of drugs with animal drug self-administration procedures: Psychomotor stimulants and hallucinogens. *Adv Behav Pharmacol*, 1979. **2**: p. 163–208.
14. Ionamin. Available from: https://www.accessdata.fda.gov/drugsatfda_docs/label/2012/011613s027lbl.pdf.
15. Lomaira. Available from: https://lomaira.com/Prescribing_Information.pdf.
16. Thomas, C.E., et al., Low adoption of weight loss medications: A comparison of prescribing patterns of antiobesity pharmacotherapies and SGLT2s. *Obesity (Silver Spring)*, 2016. **24**(9): pp. 1955–61.
17. Atkinson, R.L., et al., Long-term drug treatment of obesity in a private practice setting. *Obes Res*, 1997. **5**(6): pp. 578–86.

18. Weintraub, M., Long-term weight control: The National Heart, Lung, and Blood Institute funded multimodal intervention study. *Clin Pharmacol Ther*, 1992. **51**(5): pp. 581–5.
19. Weintraub, M., et al., A double-blind clinical trial in weight control. Use of fenfluramine and phentermine alone and in combination. *Arch Intern Med*, 1984. **144**(6): pp. 1143–8.
20. Gadde, K.M., et al., Effects of low-dose, controlled-release, phentermine plus topiramate combination on weight and associated comorbidities in overweight and obese adults (CONQUER): A randomised, placebo-controlled, phase 3 trial. *Lancet*, 2011. **377**(9774): pp. 1341–52.
21. Contrave. Available from https://www.accessdata.fda.gov/drugsatfda_docs/label/2014/200063s000lbl.pdf.
22. Apovian, C.M., et al., A randomized, phase 3 trial of naltrexone SR/bupropion SR on weight and obesity-related risk factors (COR-II). *Obesity (Silver Spring)*, 2013. **21**(5): pp. 935–43.
23. Hollander, P., et al., Effects of naltrexone sustained-release/bupropion sustained-release combination therapy on body weight and glycemic parameters in overweight and obese patients with type 2 diabetes. *Diabetes Care*, 2013. **36**(12): pp. 4022–9.
24. Greenway, F.L., et al., Effect of naltrexone plus bupropion on weight loss in overweight and obese adults (COR-I): A multicentre, randomised, double-blind, placebo-controlled, phase 3 trial. *Lancet*, 2010. **376**(9741): pp. 595–605.
25. Pi-Sunyer, X., et al., A randomized, controlled trial of 3.0 mg of liraglutide in weight management. *N Engl J Med*, 2015. **373**(1): pp. 11–22.
26. le Roux, C.W., et al., 3 years of liraglutide versus placebo for type 2 diabetes risk reduction and weight management in individuals with prediabetes: A randomised, double-blind trial. *Lancet*, 2017. **389**(10077): pp. 1399–1409.
27. Davies, M.J., et al., Efficacy of liraglutide for weight loss among patients with type 2 diabetes: The SCALE diabetes randomized clinical trial. *JAMA*, 2015. **314**(7): pp. 687–99.
28. Blackman, A., et al., Effect of liraglutide 3.0 mg in individuals with obesity and moderate or severe obstructive sleep apnea: The SCALE Sleep Apnea randomized clinical trial. *Int J Obes (Lond)*, 2016. **40**(8): pp. 1310–9.
29. Marso, S.P., et al., Liraglutide and cardiovascular outcomes in type 2 diabetes. *N Engl J Med*, 2016. **375**(4): p. 311–22.
30. Smith, S.R., et al., Lorcaserin (APD356), a selective 5-HT(2C) agonist, reduces body weight in obese men and women. *Obesity (Silver Spring)*, 2009. **17**(3): pp. 494–503.
31. Fidler, M.C., et al., A one-year randomized trial of lorcaserin for weight loss in obese and overweight adults: The BLOSSOM trial. *J Clin Endocrinol Metab*, 2011. **96**(10): pp. 3067–77.
32. Smith, S.R., et al., Multicenter, placebo-controlled trial of lorcaserin for weight management. *N Engl J Med*, 2010. **363**(3): pp. 245–256.
33. Weissman, N.J., et al., Echocardiographic assessment of cardiac valvular regurgitation with lorcaserin from analysis of 3 phase 3 clinical trials. *Circ Cardiovasc Imaging*, 2013. **6**(4): pp. 560–7.
34. Orlistat. Available from https://www.accessdata.fda.gov/drugsatfda_docs/label/2012/020766s029lbl.pdf.
35. Davidson, M.H., et al., Weight control and risk factor reduction in obese subjects treated for 2 years with orlistat: A randomized controlled trial. *JAMA*, 1999. **281**(3): pp. 235–42.
36. Hollander, P.A., et al., Role of orlistat in the treatment of obese patients with type 2 diabetes. A 1-year randomized double-blind study. *Diabetes Care*, 1998. **21**(8): pp. 1288–94.

37. Jacob, S., et al., Orlistat 120 mg improves glycaemic control in type 2 diabetic patients with or without concurrent weight loss. *Diabetes Obes Metab*, 2009. **11**(4): pp. 361–71.

38. Kristensen, M., et al., Supplementation with dairy calcium and/or flaxseed fibers in conjunction with orlistat augments fecal fat excretion without altering ratings of gastro-intestinal comfort. *Nutr Metab (Lond)*, 2017. **14**: p. 13.

39. Fildes, A., et al., Probability of an obese person attaining normal body weight: Cohort study using electronic health records. *Am J Public Health*, 2015. **105**(9): p. e54–9.

40. Kushner, R.F. and G.D. Foster, Obesity and quality of life. *Nutrition*, 2000. **16**(10): pp. 947–52.

41. Dhurandhar, N.V., et al., Predictors of weight loss outcomes in obesity care: results of the national ACTION study. *BMC Public Health*, 2019. **19**(1): p. 1422.

42. Apovian, C.M., et al., Pharmacological management of obesity: an endocrine Society clinical practice guideline. *J Clin Endocrinol Metab*, 2015. **100**(2): pp. 342–62.

43. Domecq, J.P., et al., Clinical review: Drugs commonly associated with weight change: A systematic review and meta-analysis. *J Clin Endocrinol Metab*, 2015. **100**(2): pp. 363–70.

44. Singh, A.K. and R. Singh, Pharmacotherapy in obesity: A systematic review and meta-analysis of randomized controlled trials of anti-obesity drugs. *Expert Rev Clin Pharmacol*, 2020. **13**(1): pp. 53–64.

45. Rems, Q., Available from: https://www.qsymiarems.com/.

46. Pasarica, M., et al., Collaborative learning activity utilizing evidence-based medicine to improve medical student learning of the lifestyle management of obesity. *MedEdPORTAL*, 2016. **12**: p. 10426.

47. Pasarica, M. and D. Topping, An evidence-based approach to teaching obesity management to medical students. *MedEdPORTAL*, 2017. **13**: p. 10662.

9 Bariatric Surgery

Robert F. Kushner, MD
Northwestern University Feinberg School of Medicine

CONTENTS

9.1   INTRODUCTION

As part of a comprehensive treatment plan for patients with obesity, it is important that health care professionals become familiar with the indications, procedures, complications, and management aspects of metabolic and bariatric surgery. These procedures represent an effective treatment option for patients with moderate to severe obesity – categories of patients that are seen in every medical practice. In 2018, there were approximately 252,000 bariatric procedures performed in the United States [1]. Health care professionals from all disciplines need to recognize eligible candidates for surgery and know how to monitor and manage these patients on a long-term basis. Thus, this chapter is intended as a primer on the most commonly performed weight loss procedures, the importance of preoperative and postoperative management, identification and management of nutritional deficiencies that may occur following bariatric surgery, and factors associated with weight regain.

9.2   BARIATRIC SURGICAL PROCEDURES

Weight loss surgeries have traditionally been classified into three categories on the basis of anatomic changes: restrictive, restrictive malabsorptive, and malabsorptive (Figure 9.1). More recently, however, the clinical benefits of bariatric surgery in achieving weight loss and alleviating metabolic comorbidities have been attributed largely to changes in the physiologic responses of gut hormones, bile acid metabolism, microbiota, and adipose tissue metabolism [2] (Figures 9.2 and 9.3).

9.2.1   RESTRICTIVE SURGERIES

Restrictive surgeries limit the amount of food the stomach can hold and slow the rate of gastric emptying. The Laparoscopic Adjustable Gastric Banding (LAGB) is the prototype of this category. The diameter of these bands is adjustable by way of

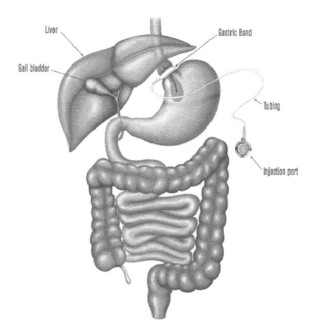

FIGURE 9.1   Adjustable gastric band. (©Ethicon, Inc. 2021. Reproduced with permission.)

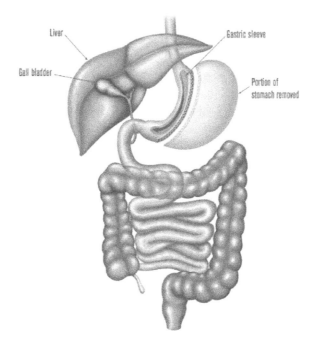

FIGURE 9.2 Vertical sleeve gastrectomy. (©Ethicon, Inc. 2021. Reproduced with permission.)

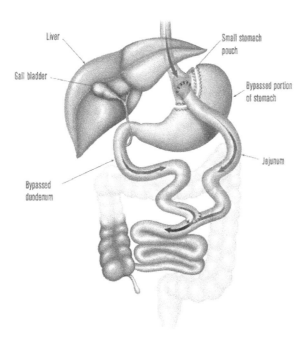

FIGURE 9.3 Roux-en-Y gastric bypass. (©Ethicon, Inc. 2021. Reproduced with permission.)

its connection to a reservoir that is implanted under the skin. Injection or removal of saline into the reservoir tightens or loosens the band's internal diameter, respectively, thus changing the size of the gastric opening. Since there is no rerouting of the intestine with LAGB, the risk for developing nutritional deficiencies is entirely dependent on the patient's diet and eating habits. However, due to poor long-term weight loss response, the LAGB has fallen into disfavor and accounts for <2% of all bariatric surgeries performed [1]. The most commonly performed procedure (accounting for 61% of all procedures) is the laparoscopic sleeve gastrectomy (SG). In this procedure, the stomach is restricted by stapling and dividing it vertically and removing approximately 80% of the greater curvature, leaving a slim "banana-shaped" remnant stomach along the lesser curvature.

9.2.2 RESTRICTIVE MALABSORPTIVE BYPASS PROCEDURE

The restrictive malabsorptive bypass procedure combines the elements of gastric restriction with limited macronutrient malabsorption, primarily of fat. The prototype procedure is the Roux-en-Y Gastric Bypass (RYGB) (accounting for 17% of all procedures). A 10- to 30-ml proximal gastric pouch is formed by surgically separating the stomach across the fundus. Outflow from the pouch is created by performing a narrow (10 mm) gastrojejunostomy. The distal end of jejunum is then anastomosed 50–150 cm below the gastrojejunostomy. "Roux-en-Y" refers to the Y-shaped section of small intestine created by the surgery; the Y is created at the point where the pancreo-biliary conduit (afferent limb) and the Roux (efferent) limb are connected. "Bypass" refers to the exclusion or bypassing of the distal stomach, duodenum, and proximal jejunum. The biliopancreatic diversion with duodenal switch (BPD/DS), a malabsorptive procedure, is uncommonly performed and will not be discussed further. The remaining 15% of all bariatric procedures are revisional re-operations.

9.3 WHY CONSIDER BARIATRIC SURGERY? LONG-TERM OUTCOMES AND RESOLUTION OF COMORBID CONDITIONS

9.3.1 WEIGHT LOSS OUTCOMES

Although specific patient outcomes may vary, bariatric surgery is the most effective approach for weight loss and treatment of comorbid conditions. In a meta-analysis of 11 randomized controlled trials, mean BMI reduction was 13.5 kg/m^2 for RYGB, 14.4 kg/m^2 for SG, and 10.6 kg/m^2 for LAGB [3]. The trajectory of weight loss also differs between procedure types. Whereas the rate of weight loss is slower with LAGB, with maximal weight loss achieved after 2 or 3 years, maximal weight loss with RYGB and SG is achieved at 12–18 months. In the Longitudinal Assessment of Bariatric Surgery (LABS) study, a prospective observational study of about 2,500 patients who underwent bariatric surgery, median nadir (maximum) weight loss was 37.4% (25th –75th % = 14%–39%) of preoperative weight [4]. Longer-term weight loss was analyzed in a prospective study by Adams et al. who followed over 400 patients who underwent the RYGB procedure, with greater than 90% follow-up at 12 years. At year 12, compared to baseline, 93% maintained at least 10% total weight loss, 70%

maintained at least a 20% weight loss, and 40% maintained at least a 30% weight loss. In contrast, control patients did not experience significant weight loss over the 12-year follow-up period [5].

9.3.2 MEDICAL OUTCOMES

The combined effects of significant weight loss and surgically induced metabolic changes lead to established improvement in multiple obesity-related comorbid conditions including type 2 diabetes (T2D), hypertension, dyslipidemia, and obstructive sleep apnea [4–8]. One of the most important clinical outcomes is the role of bariatric surgery in the treatment of patients with T2D. A substantial body of evidence demonstrates that metabolic and bariatric surgery achieves superior glycemic control in patients with T2D compared with various medical and lifestyle interventions [8]. The improvement in diabetes control appears to be due to both weight loss and weight loss independent effects [9]. Based on these data, the Second Diabetes Surgery Summit (DSS-II) Consensus Conference published guidelines in 2015 that were endorsed by more than 50 other organizations interested in the treatment of diabetes [10]. According to the guidelines, metabolic and bariatric surgery should be recommended to treat T2D in patients with class II obesity when hyperglycemia is inadequately controlled with lifestyle and optimal medical therapy and should be similarly considered for those with class I obesity (BMI 30.0–34.9 kg/m^2). The 2020 Standards of Care for the treatment of diabetes from the American Diabetes Association includes bariatric surgery in the treatment algorithm [11].

9.4 SELECTING THE APPROPRIATE PATIENT

Patients with severe class III obesity (BMI $\geq$ 40 kg/m^2) or moderate class II obesity (BMI 35–39.9 kg/m^2) with obesity-related comorbidities (e.g. diabetes, obstructive sleep apnea, hypertension) are candidates for bariatric surgery if they have not responded to behavioral treatment (with or without pharmacotherapy) with sufficient weight loss to achieve health outcome goals [12]. Despite demonstrated benefit in patients with class 1 obesity (30–34.9 kg/m^2) and inadequately controlled diabetes, few insurance companies in the US will approve surgery for this category. Contraindications to surgery are listed in Table 9.1.

When broaching the topic of bariatric surgery with patients, it is important to assess their knowledge and concerns, provide additional resources (e.g. websites, handouts, or information on orientation sessions) and refer to an experienced metabolic and bariatric center. Most centers employ (or have access to) a multidisciplinary team that includes medical providers, a registered dietitian nutritionist (RDN), health psychologist, and bariatric surgeon.

9.5 EVALUATING AND PREPARING THE PATIENT FOR SURGERY

All patients who are considering weight loss surgery should undergo a comprehensive medical, psychological, and nutritional assessment. Clinical Practice Guidelines for the perioperative nutrition, metabolic, and nonsurgical support of patients

TABLE 9.1

Contraindications for Bariatric Surgery

- Uncontrolled mental health disorder (e.g. major depressive disorder, bipolar disorder, schizophrenia, acute psychosis, suicidal ideation)
- Active substance abuse (drugs/alcohol)
- Uncontrolled eating disorder (e.g. bulimia nervosa)
- Unwilling to adhere with necessary guidelines following bariatric surgery
- Hormonal causes of obesity that can be medically treated (e.g. Cushing disease)
- Severe cardiopulmonary disease
- Terminal cancer

undergoing bariatric procedures are available to guide this process [13]. Preparation for surgery may span 6 months depending on the patient's medical condition and requirements for insurance approval.

9.5.1 Medical Evaluation

Depending on the bariatric center, preoperative medical evaluation and treatment of risk factors may be conducted by the primary care provider or the bariatric surgery center. The goal is to optimize the patient's health and modify risk factors to ensure surgery is performed under optimal conditions. A complete history and physical examination is performed to identify obesity-related comorbidities and indications for surgery. Cardiology evaluations for risk assessment should follow standards of practice for perioperative evaluation and management of patients undergoing noncardiac surgery. Patients with significant snoring, witnessed apnea episodes, morning headaches, or daytime sleepiness should be screened for obstructive sleep apnea (OSA) and prescribed continuous positive airway pressure (CPAP) treatment to optimize their pulmonary status for at least 1 month prior to surgery. Some centers routinely obtain esophagogastroduodenoscopy (EGD) on all patients, while others are more selective and perform preoperative EGDs only when indicated, such as a history of dyspepsia, reflux, dysphagia, or previous ulcer disease.

Routine laboratory tests typically include a comprehensive metabolic profile (CMP) and complete blood count (CBC), lipid profile, thyroid function, urinalysis, prothrombin time/INR, blood type, and micronutrient screening that includes iron studies, ferritin, vitamin B_{12}, folic acid, 25-OH vitamin D, and iPTH [13]. The nutrient screening is essential to uncover any deficiencies that need to be corrected prior to surgery. Although the literature is conflicting regarding the benefit of mandating preoperative weight loss as a criterion to undergo surgery, it is reasonable to include modest preoperative weight loss as an expectation during the preoperative period.

9.5.2 Psychological Evaluation

The psychological evaluation is an insurance requirement and typically performed by a psychologist affiliated with the bariatric surgery center. The primary purpose is to assess the patient's psychosocial functioning, health behaviors and coping patterns, and presence of any underlying eating or psychiatric disorders that may worsen or impair the bariatric surgical process and outcomes. Patients who are identified with problematic psychosocial, behavioral, or psychiatric issues are often asked to attend a limited number of counseling sessions to address these concerns preoperatively.

9.5.3 NUTRITIONAL EVALUATION

The nutritional evaluation is typically performed by an RDN affiliated with the bariatric surgery center to determine if the patient meets the medically accepted criteria for bariatric surgery, educate the patient on potential health benefits and risks of surgery, and determine the patient's ability to incorporate nutritional and behavioral changes. The RDN also evaluates the patient's current diet, past weight loss attempts, nutritional deficiencies, or any disordered eating patterns including triggers to weight gain or challenges to following a healthy diet.

9.5.4 PREPARING THE PATIENT FOR SURGERY

During the preoperative process, patients are typically counseled by the bariatric surgical team on healthy eating and physical activity patterns, behavioral strategies to implement the lifestyle changes, and the importance of stress reduction and social support for long-term success. Specific dietary and nutritional recommendations pertinent to the surgical procedures include use of protein supplements, consumption of multiple meals and snacks, and slowing the rate of eating. Patients are seen either individually or in small groups. Many centers offer panel discussions between candidate patients and patients who have already undergone a procedure to provide a peer-to-peer discussion of risks, benefits, and challenges of life after bariatric surgery.

9.6 POSTOPERATIVE CARE

9.6.1 IMMEDIATE MANAGEMENT (<3 MONTHS)

Perioperative mortality rates for bariatric surgery range from 0.03% to 0.2%; comparable rates for cholecystectomy or hip replacement are 0.7% and 0.93%, respectively [14]. Similarly, the 30-day risk of serious adverse events (such as reoperation, prolonged hospitalization, and venous thromboembolism) is generally less than 6%. Patients are typically discharged after 1–2 days and counseled on a dietary plan that is slowly advanced over the first 4–6 weeks. They are also instructed to take two chewable multiple vitamin-mineral supplements daily.

Medication adjustments are commonly made immediately upon discharge. For patients with T2D, the use of all insulin secretagogues (sulfonylureas and meglitinides), sodium-glucose cotransporter-2 inhibitors, and thiazolidinediones should be discontinued and insulin doses adjusted (due to low-calorie intake) to minimize the risk for hypoglycemia. Except for metformin and incretin-based therapies, antidiabetic medications should be withheld if there is no evidence of hyperglycemia. Metformin and/or incretin-based therapies may be continued postoperatively in patients with T2D until prolonged clinical resolution of T2D is demonstrated by normalized glycemic targets [13,15]. For patients with hypertension, diuretic agents should be discontinued to avoid dehydration, hypotension, and electrolyte abnormalities. Due to the increased risk of postoperative ulcers, strictures, and bleeding, the chronic use of nonsteroidal anti-inflammatory drugs (NSAIDS) should be avoided in RYGB patients. Decisions on continued use of antidepressants, antilipidemic medications, and other categories of medications should be determined on an individual basis.

9.6.2 SURGICAL AND MEDICAL EMERGENCIES

Patients should be referred to the bariatric center or emergency department for urgent evaluation for any immediate concerns during the initial postoperative period. Signs of a potential emergency include tachycardia which is the first sign of a potential leak, fever >101.5°F, dyspnea, chest pain, leg pain and swelling, persistent nausea and vomiting, or intolerance to oral intake. Nausea and vomiting are symptoms that warrant particular attention and can occur following any of the bariatric surgery procedures. Although most commonly unrelated to obstruction or anatomical defect of the surgery, if the patient is not able to keep anything down by mouth for 24 hours, an evaluation is warranted. One important sequela of persistent nausea and vomiting is Wernicke's encephalopathy [16]. This is the most significant medical emergency that must be urgently treated to avoid an irreversible neurologic pontine stroke. Patients with persistent vomiting may deplete their thiamine stores in just a few days. The signs and symptoms of thiamine deficiency (Wernicke's) are:

- Ataxia (unsteady gait)
- Nystagmus (repetitive, uncontrolled movements of the eyes)
- Mental confusion (disoriented, hard time focusing, or making decisions)

Depending on the severity of deficiency, treatment should consist of:

- Intravenous (IV) administration of 200mg of thiamine three times per day or
- Oral administration 500mg once or twice daily for three to five consecutive days followed by 250mg for the next 3–5days, or
- Intramuscular (IM) administration of 250mg daily for 3–5days or 100–150 monthly.

Once the patient can tolerate oral intake, 100mg of thiamine supplementation is recommended for at least 30days.

9.7 LONG-TERM MANAGEMENT

9.7.1 MEDICAL MANAGEMENT

As patients continue to lose weight over the first 1–3 years, they need ongoing management of their existing comorbid conditions, may require adjustment of medications and other prescribed treatments, and may require monitoring of their nutritional status. Continued monitoring of T2D is particularly required since as many as one-third of RYGB patients and 42% of sleeve patients who initially experience remission of T2D eventually relapse [8]. People with earlier-stage T2D (i.e. did not need insulin preoperatively, shorter duration of disease, and lower HbA1c) appear to have a longer remission rate. Other preexisting medical problems, such as osteoarthritis, gastroesophageal reflux disease, urinary incontinence, asthma, heart disease, and hyperlipidemia, should be managed according to symptoms or laboratory values [13]. Patients with obstructive sleep apnea will frequently experience an improvement in sleep quality and reduction in the apnea hypopnea index (AHI). A repeat sleep study and re-titration of CPAP is often performed 6–12 months postoperatively

9.7.2 Nutritional Management

It is important that all patients who undergo bariatric surgery have periodic visits with an RDN for dietary counseling. This is most commonly arranged through the bariatric center.

As a result of the reductions in gastric capacity and caloric intake after surgery, patients must take care to ensure that nutritional needs are met. Postoperative patients are advised to consume small portions, have 4–6 small meals daily, and ensure an adequate intake of lean protein (60–120 g/day), fruits and vegetables (>5 servings/day), and whole grains [13]. Patients are instructed to eat slowly, chew thoroughly, avoid fatty foods, sweets and sugar-sweetened beverages, and avoid ingestion of liquids within 30 minutes of meals.

Food intolerances may occur after surgery that lead to alterations in dietary patterns. Lactose intolerance can develop in patients who have undergone RYGB; as a result, nearly one-third of patients report avoiding milk after the procedure. Dumping syndrome (a clinical condition caused by rapid gastric emptying of concentrated sugar into the small intestine) occurs in up to three-quarters of patients after RYGB and is associated with postprandial symptoms, such as abdominal cramping, nausea, diarrhea, lightheadedness, sweating, and tachycardia [13]. Dumping syndrome can usually be managed by dietary modification, including avoidance of concentrated sweets and simple sugars, consumption of small frequent meals, and inclusion of protein at every meal.

Patients with symptoms suggestive of postprandial hypoglycemia that are not ameliorated by dietary modification should undergo evaluation for the presence of hyperinsulinemic hypoglycemia, particularly when associated with more severe neuroglycopenic symptoms, such as confusion or loss of consciousness [17]. For most patients with post-bypass hypoglycemia, dietary modification, including carbohydrate restriction to less than 30 g per meal, can significantly reduce the frequency and severity of symptoms. However, when symptoms persist, pharmacologic therapies, such as acarbose, diazoxide, somatostatin analogs, and calcium channel blockers, may be required. Patients with hyperinsulinemic hypoglycemia should be referred to an endocrinologist or the bariatric surgery center for further evaluation and treatment.

Patients who have undergone bariatric surgery need to be followed for the rest of their life for the prevention and management of micronutrient (microminerals and vitamins) deficiencies that are the result of the surgical anatomical changes. After RYGB, the most common micronutrient deficiencies include those of iron, vitamin B_{12}, vitamin D, and calcium [13]. Folic acid deficiency has also been reported but is largely preventable with regular use of a standard multivitamin preparation. Sleeve gastrectomy has been reported to produce similar deficiencies as gastric bypass but at a somewhat lower frequency. Purely restrictive procedures such as LAGB are infrequently associated with specific nutritional deficiencies.

In most cases, micronutrient deficiencies can be prevented by regular vitamin and mineral supplementation along with appropriate clinical follow up and routine biochemical surveillance. Expert guidelines are available regarding recommended vitamin and mineral supplementation after surgery and the frequency of laboratory screening for deficiency states [13,15,18]. Tables 9.2 and 9.3 summarize these recommendations. Patients who are found to have evidence of specific micronutrient deficiencies will need additional vitamin or mineral supplementation, as indicated.

9.7.2.1 Iron

Iron deficiency is more commonly found after RYGB since it is most efficiently absorbed in the duodenum and proximal jejunum, which is bypassed following this procedure [19]. Malabsorption of iron coincides with a decreased intake of iron-containing foods such as red meats, grains, and vegetables. Menstruating women or those with menorrhagia are at particularly high risk. Iron deficiency is the

---

TABLE 9.2

Recommended Laboratory Tests and Frequency of Routine Biochemical Surveillance

Micronutrient	Supplementation to Prevent Deficiency	Repletion for Patients with Deficiency
Vitamin B1[a] (thiamine)	≥12 mg daily, preferably 50 mg from a B-complex supplement	Oral therapy: 100 mg 2–3 times daily IV therapy: 200 mg 3 times daily for 3–5 days, followed by 250 mg/day for 3–5 days
Vitamin B12	Orally: 350–1,000 mcg daily Nasal spray: as directed by manufacturer Parenteral (IM or SC): 1,000 mcg monthly	1,000 mcg/day to achieve normal levels
Folate[a]	400–800 mg oral daily	Oral dose of 1,000 mg daily to achieve normal levels
Iron[a]	18–60 mg elemental iron/day	150–300 mg elemental iron/day in divided doses
Calcium	1,200–1,500 mg/day	1,800–2,400 mg/day
Vitamin D	3,000 IU/day	3,000–6,000 IU vitamin D3/day 50,000 IU vitamin D2, 1–3 times weekly
Vitamin A[a]	5,000–10,000 IU/day	10,000–25,000 IU/day

Adapted from Ref. [13].

[a] typically consumed in a multivitamin plus mineral supplement.

TABLE 9.3

Nutritional Supplementation and Repletion after Bariatric Surgery

	LABG	SG	RYGB
Timing	Every 6 months in the first year	Every 3–6 months in the first year	Every 3–6 months in the first year
	Every 12 months thereafter	Every 12 months thereafter	Every 12 months thereafter
Assessment	CBC, platelets, electrolytes, iron, ferritin, vitamin B12, folate, vitamin D, PTH	CBC, platelets, electrolytes, iron, ferritin, vitamin B12, folate, vitamin D, PTH	CBC, platelets, electrolytes, iron, ferritin, vitamin B12, folate, vitamin D, PTH, 24-hour urinary calcium, osteocalcin

Adapted from Ref. [15].

LAGB, laparoscopic adjustable gastric banding; RYGB, SG, sleeve gastrectomy Roux-en-Y gastric bypass; CBC, complete blood count; PTH, parathyroid hormone.

main cause of anemia for bariatric surgery patients but anemia may also result from low levels of vitamin B_{12} and folate. Symptoms may include fatigue and reduced capacity for exercise tolerance. To prevent iron deficiency, all patients should be evaluated prior to surgery to determine any pre-existing diminished iron stores.

9.7.2.2 Vitamin B_{12}

Malabsorptive and restrictive bariatric surgical procedures interfere with several key processes of vitamin B_{12} absorption. Due to changes in hydrochloric acid (HCl) production and reduced availability of intrinsic factor (IF), B_{12} absorption is impaired [16]. Post-RYGB, patients no longer have the ability to release vitamin B_{12} from protein foods because pepsinogen cannot be converted into pepsin due to the lack of HCl. Decreased production of IF by the parietal cells in the stomach will also prevent vitamin B_{12} from being absorbed. The parietal cells that excrete acid and IF, as well as the cells that excrete pepsinogen, are located primarily in the fundus and body of the stomach and are bypassed after RYGB.

If not supplemented, patients may begin to exhibit signs and symptoms of B_{12} deficiency which include macrocytic anemia, glossitis, numbness or tingling in the lower extremities, changes in gait or motor skills, loss of concentration, memory loss, or disorientation. Serum B_{12} levels alone, especially when at the lower end of the normal range, may be inadequate to diagnosis deficiency. Elevated methylmalonic acid (MMA) level is a better test since it is specific for metabolic changes seen in vitamin B_{12} deficiency.

9.7.2.3 Calcium and Vitamin D

Calcium and Vitamin D are typically grouped, as a deficiency in one or both of these may lead to metabolic bone disease, increased bone turnover, secondary hyperparathyroidism (HPT), undermineralized bone, and bone loss [20]. As reduction in bone mineral density and bone mineral content generally accompanies weight loss, it is crucial to differentiate between the effects of weight loss compared to the malabsorptive consequences of bariatric surgery. A deficiency of calcium and vitamin D may result from a decrease in calcium and vitamin D-rich dairy foods related to intolerance, or by a reduction in intestinal absorption resulting from surgical bypass of the duodenum and proximal jejunum. Calcium is absorbed in the duodenum and proximal jejunum and is dependent on vitamin D levels. Vitamin D is absorbed in the small intestine, which is altered following RYGB. Although calcium and vitamin D deficiencies are more prevalent in patients undergoing malabsoprtive procedures, patients who had SG and LAGB can still experience calcium and vitamin D deficiencies due to poor food intake, usually related to intolerances to dairy products.

While calcium and vitamin D deficiency following malabsorptive procedures is predictable, patients often present with unrecognized deficiencies preoperatively. Patients with a high BMI may be subject to develop vitamin D deficiencies related to decreased bioavailability of vitamin D due to enhanced uptake and clearance by adipose tissues, or underexposure to the sun. Patients with severe obesity should be screened for vitamin D deficiency and abnormalities in bone density prior to bariatric surgery. Periodic measurements of 25 (OH) vitamin D, PTH, and calcium should be obtained prior to and periodically after surgery.

9.7.3 RECOMMENDATIONS FOR PHYSICAL ACTIVITY AFTER BARIATRIC SURGERY

National guidelines suggest that for optimal weight control, most individuals who are overweight will need to accumulate at least 150–300 minutes of moderate physical activity per week, or 30–60 minutes most days of the week [21]. Other data from the National Weight Control Registry indicate that walking is the preferred form of physical activity in this group of individuals [22]. In randomized controlled trials as well as epidemiologic studies, individuals who use pedometers to reach a specific step-count goal (such as >10,000 steps/day) increase their activity levels more and lose slightly more weight than those who do not use pedometers [23]. In addition, since bariatric surgery leads to loss of lean body mass, patients should be counseled to incorporate strength training exercises at least twice weekly to preserve muscle mass.

9.7.4 PSYCHOLOGICAL CARE

Bariatric surgical patients experience a variety of psychosocial challenges in the postoperative period. Initially, patients must adjust to the postoperative diet and to their altered relationship with food. As weight loss progresses, patients must adapt to changes in their appearance and their interactions with others. Dramatic weight loss, however desirable to the patient, can lead to unexpected consequences, such as body image issues related to excess skin, unwanted sexual attention from others, and jealousy from friends and loved ones. As a result of these many challenges, screening for mood disorders and substance abuse is important among postoperative patients.

Patients who have undergone bariatric surgery may be at an increased risk of suicide, particularly in the first 3 years after surgery. In one large retrospective cohort study, individuals who had undergone gastric bypass surgery were twice as likely to commit suicide as control subjects with obesity matched for sex, age, and baseline BMI [24]. Case studies suggest that patients who commit suicide after bariatric surgery often have a history of recurrent major depression, both before and after surgery, and that their depression persists even if they have excellent weight loss results. These reports highlight the importance of continued attention to psychosocial health in the postoperative period, regardless of weight loss outcomes.

Several prospective studies have demonstrated an increased prevalence of alcohol use disorder (AUD) up to 7-years postoperatively. In a sub-study of LABS, patients completed baseline and follow-up assessments of alcohol consumption using the Alcohol Use Disorders Identification Test (AUDIT), a 10-item test. After RYGB, there was an increase in the prevalence of AUD at baseline (pre-surgery) (6.6%) to year 2 (9.6%) and year 7 (16.4%) [25]. In another comprehensive review of the literature [26], a preoperative history of substance use (including alcohol) was a reliable predictor of postoperative use.

9.8   WEIGHT REGAIN FOLLOWING BARIATRIC SURGERY

Although bariatric surgery is considered the most effective treatment for obesity, it is not a cure. Weight regain can occur following all the bariatric procedures and needs to be monitored at every office visit. Follow up data from the LABS study has continued to inform clinical care regarding various aspects of postoperative management, including postoperative weight loss trajectories [27], and predictors of weight change [28], The underlying factors that influence weight regain following bariatric surgery are multifactorial and include the biological forces that defend body weight, dietary indiscretion, mental health issues, physical inactivity, and rarely, anatomic surgical failure. The extent and significance of these factors are currently uncertain and likely vary between individuals and the operative procedure performed. Five-year observational data from the LABS study shows that median weight regain was 25.2% of maximum weight loss (25th% – 75th% = 14%–39%) [29]. Thus, some weight gain is a normal and expected outcome from bariatric surgery and commonly leads to patient distress and frustration. The LABS study also showed that recurrence of diabetes, hypertension, and dyslipidemia along with worsening quality of life outcomes was associated with weight regain. Table 9.4 provides a categorical list of potential causes that should be explored with all patients who present with weight regain [30]. Depending on the patient's age and gender, a thorough history should be performed that reviews all of these reasons followed by appropriate counseling.

Similar to any patient who presents with unintentional weight gain, it is important to screen for prescription of weight gaining medications (e.g. insulin, sulfonylureas, some psychotropic and antidepressant drugs, steroids), onset of new medical problems (e.g. hypothyroidism), and occurrence of life events that impact diet, physical activity, or mental health. Disruption of the surgery is the least likely cause but should be considered in patients who no longer feel dietary restraint. In this select group, initial evaluation consists of ordering an upper GI x-ray or EGD. Surgical interventions may include conversion of an SG to a RYGB, or endoscopic procedures that are designed to tighten the gastric pouch or anastomosis. Consultation with the bariatric center or a trained gastroenterologist is warranted if these procedures are considered. Essentially all patients will benefit from seeing an RDN for dietary counseling. Referral to a health psychologist should be considered for patients who

TABLE 9.4

Etiological Factors for Weight Regain Following Bariatric Surgery [30]

Anatomical
  LAGB malfunction or mismanagement
  Band or port breakage, band too loose
  RYGB
  Pouch enlargement
  Gastrojejunal anastomosis dilation
  Gastro-gastro fistula
Physiological
  Pregnancy
  Menopause
  Medications which cause weight gain
  Smoking cessation
  Endocrine disorders: hypothyroidism, Cushing's syndrome, insulinoma
  Intestinal or hormonal adaptation
Behavioral
  Dietary
  Unhealthy eating patterns, e.g. grazing, nibbling, mindless eating
  Consumption of energy-dense foods and beverages
  Loss of dumping syndrome symptoms
  Loss of control over urges, binges
  Reduced vigilance
  Physical activity
  Reduced leisure time activity
  Increased sedentary behaviors
  Insufficient moderately and vigorously intensity exercise
  Development of physical limitations to exercise

are struggling with making behavioral changes, developed substance misuse, or have any mental health disorders.

Although there is limited data regarding the use of anti-obesity medications (AOM) for patients who experience weight regain or inadequate weight loss following bariatric surgery, this is a rational and practical treatment that will continue to emerge. Four AOMs that control appetite are currently approved by the Food and Drug Administration (FDA) for chronic weight management in patients with a BMI $\geq$30 kg/m^2 or $\geq$27 with a weight-related comorbidity. These include phentermine/topiramate (Qsymia®), naltrexone/bupropion (Contrave®), liraglutide 3.0 mg (Saxenda®) and semaglutide 2.4 mg (Wegovy®). All of the studies of AOM use after bariatric surgery to date have been uncontrolled, observational, and retrospective analyses of single- or multicenter cohorts who received one of multiple AOMs [31]. Although the timing, duration, and selection of medications varied widely, a clinically significant response ($\geq$5% weight loss) was seen across all studies. The use of adjunctive pharmacotherapy is a reasonable approach and should follow current prescription guidelines.

9.9 CONCLUSION

Bariatric surgery is an effective and acceptable treatment for individuals with moderate or severe obesity who are at risk for or have complications associated with obesity. Several surgical procedures are available with variable risk and weight loss outcomes. However, regardless of the procedure performed, surgery is considered a tool that is adjunctive to choosing a healthy, calorie-controlled diet and engaging in daily physical activity. For patients who undergo a restrictive-malabsorptive operation, micronutrient supplementation is necessary to avoid nutritional deficiencies. Patients are at risk for weight regain following surgery due to several biopsychosocial factors. In order to maximize successful outcomes, all patients should be monitored and managed by a multidisciplinary team of health care providers knowledgeable in bariatric surgical care.

PRACTICAL APPLICATIONS

- In the discussion of treatment options for patients with moderate and severe obesity, it is important that health care professionals become familiar with the indications, procedures, complications, and management aspects of metabolic and bariatric surgery
- Since obesity is a chronic disease without cure, health care professionals must be prepared to manage their bariatric surgery patients long-term
- In most cases, micronutrient deficiencies can be prevented by regular vitamin and mineral supplementation along with appropriate clinical follow up and routine biochemical surveillance
- Some weight regain is an expected outcome and should be thoroughly evaluated and treated on an ongoing basis

REFERENCES

1. American Society for Metabolic and Bariatric Surgery. Estimate of Bariatric Surgery Numbers, 2011–2018 https://asmbs.org/resources/estimate-of-bariatric-surgery-numbers. Accessed December 13, 2020.
2. Pucci, A., Batterham, R.L. 2019. Mechanisms underlying the weight loss effects of RYGB and SG: similar, yet different. *J Endocrinol Invest.* 42(2):117–128.
3. Kang, J.H., Jenny, H., Le, Q.A., Quang, A. 2017. Effectiveness of bariatric surgical procedures. A systematic review and network meta-analysis of randomized controlled trials. *Medicine* 96(46):e8632.
4. Courcoulas, A.P., King, W.C., Belle, S.H., et al. 2018. Seven-year weight trajectories and health outcomes in the longitudinal assessment of bariatric surgery (LABS) study. *JAMA Surg* 153(5):427–434.
5. Adams, T.D., Davidson, L.E., Litwin, S.E., et al. 2017. Weight and metabolic outcomes 12 years after gastric bypass. *N Engl J Med* 377(12):1143–1155.
6. Poirier, P., Cornier, M.A., Mazzone, T., et al. 2011. Bariatric surgery and cardiovascular risk factors: A scientific statement from the American Heart Association. *Circulation* 123(15):1683–1701.
7. Kwok, C.S., Pradhan, A., Khan, M.A., et al. 2014. Bariatric surgery and its impact on cardiovascular disease and mortality: a systematic review and meta-analysis. *Int J Cardiol* 173:20–28.

8. Arterburn, D.E., Telem, D.A., Kushner, R.F., Courcoulas, A.P. 2020 Benefits and risks of bariatric surgery in adults. *JAMA* 324(9):879–887.
9. Madsbad, S., Dirksen, C., Holst, J.J. 2014. Mechanisms of changes in glucose metabolism and bodyweight after bariatric surgery. *Lancet Diabetes Endocrinol.* 2:152–164.
10. Rubino, F., Nathan, D.M., Eckel, R.H., et al. 2016. Metabolic surgery in the treatment algorithm for type 2 diabetes. *Diabetes Care* 39(6):861–872.
11. American Diabetes Association. 2020. Obesity management for treatment of type 2 diabetes: Standards of medical care in diabetes – 2020. *Diabetes Care* 43(Supplement 1):S89–S97.
12. Jensen, M.D., Ryan, D.H., Apovian, C.M., et al. 2014. AHA/ACC/TOS guidelines for the management of overweight and obesity is adults: A report of the American College of Cardiology/American Heart Association task force on practice guidelines and The Obesity Society. *Circulation* 129(25 Suppl 2):S102–38.
13. Mechanick, J.I., Apovian, C., Brethauer, S., et al. 2020. Clinical practice guidelines for the perioperative nutrition, metabolic, and nonsurgical support of patients undergoing bariatric procedures -2019 Update: Cosponsored by American association of clinical endocrinologists/American college of endocrinology, The obesity society, American society for metabolic and bariatric surgery, obesity medicine association, and American society of anesthesiologists. *Obesity* 28(4):O1–O58. doi:10.1002/oby.22719.
14. Aminian, A., Brethauer, S.A., Kirwan, J.P., Kashyap, S.R., Burguera, B., Schauer, P.R. 2015 How safe is metabolic/diabetes surgery? *Diabetes Obes Metab* 17(2):198–201.
15. Busetto, L., Dicker, D., Azran, C., et al. 2017. Practical recommendations of the obesity management task force of the European Association for the study of obesity for the post-bariatric surgery medical management. *Obes Facts* 10:597–632.
16. Kumar, N. 2015. Neurological disorders. In *Nutrition and Bariatric Surgery*, eds. R.F. Kushner, and C.D. Still, 99–128. New York: CRC Press.
17. Salehi, M., Vella, A., McLaughlin, T., Patti, M. 2018. Hypoglycemia after gastric bypass surgery: Current concepts and controversies. *J Clin Endocrinol Metab* 103:2815–2826.
18. Parrott, J., Frank, L., Rabena, R., Craggs-Dino, L., Isom, K.A., Greiman, L. 2017. American society for metabolic and bariatric surgery integrated health nutritional guidelines for the surgical weight loss patient 2016 update: Micronutrients. *Surg Obes Relat Dis* 13(5):727–741.
19. Marinella, M.A. 2015. Anemia and bariatric surgery. In *Nutrition and Bariatric Surgery*, eds. R.F. Kushner, and C.D. Still, 61–76. New York: CRC Press.
20. Deivert, S.F., Still, C.D. 2015. Metabolic bone disease following bariatric surgery. In *Nutrition and Bariatric Surgery*, eds. R.F. Kushner, and C.D. Still, 77–98. New York: CRC Press.
21. U.S. Department of Health and Human Services. Physical Activity Guidelines for Americans, 2nd edition. Washington, DC: U.S. Department of Health and Human Services; 2018.
22. Catenacci, V.A., Ogden, L.G., Stuht, J., et al. 2007. Physical activity patterns in the National Weight Control Registry. *Obesity* 16(1): 153–161.
23. Bravata, D.M., Smith-Spangler, C., Sundaram, V., et al. 2007. Using pedometers to increase physical activity and improve health. *JAMA* 298(19): 2296–2304.
24. Adams, T.D., Gress, R.E., Smith, S.C., et al. 2007 Long-term mortality after gastric bypass surgery. *N Engl J Med* 357(8):753–761.
25. King, W.C., Chen, J.Y., Courcoulas, A.P., et al. 2017. Alcohol and other substance use after bariatric surgery: Prospective evidence from a U.S. multicenter cohort study. *Surg Obes Relat Dis* 13:1392–1404.
26. Li, L., Wu, L.T. 2016. Substance use after bariatric surgery: A review. *J Psychiatr Res* 76:16–29.

27. Courcoulas, A.P., Chirstian, N.J., Belle, S.H., et al. 2013. Weight change and health outcomes at 3 years after bariatric surgery among individuals with severe obesity. *JAMA* 310:2416–2425.
28. Mitchell, J.E., Christian, N.J., Flum, D.R., et al. 2016. Postoperative behavioral variables and weight change 3 years after bariatric surgery. *JAMA Surg* 151:752–757.
29. Courcoulas, A.P., King, W.C., Belle, S.H., et al. 2018. Seven-year weight trajectories and health outcomes in the longitudinal assessment of bariatric surgery (LABS) study. *JAMA Surg* 153(5):427–434.
30. Kushner, R.F., Sorensen, K.W. 2015. Prevention of weight regain following bariatric surgery. *Curr Obes Rep* 4:198–206.
31. Stanford, F.C., Alfaris, N., Gomez, G., et al. 2017. The utility of weight loss medications after bariatric surgery for weight regain or inadequate weight loss: A multi-center study. *Surg Obes Relat Dis* 13:491–501.

10 Pediatric Obesity

James M. Rippe, MD
Rippe Lifestyle Institute
University of Massachusetts Medical School

CONTENTS

10.1   INTRODUCTION

Childhood obesity represents a chronic disease epidemic with both medical and public health implications. The prevalence of childhood obesity has increased significantly since the 1980s, paralleling the increase of obesity in adults over the same period [1,2]. The prevalence of 2–19 year olds with obesity in the United States is 18.5% and has continued to rise over the past two decades across all age groups [3]. Childhood obesity disproportionately affects black, Hispanic, and other minority youth. Comorbid conditions, such as type 2 diabetes (T2DM), are now being increasingly diagnosed in children and are projected to increase dramatically as generations of children with obesity carry obesity into adulthood.

There has been a lag in responding to this emerging epidemic in the United States both with regard to clinical care and also medical education [4]. Many practicing clinicians feel that they lack adequate training and possess inadequate clinical background and skills for weight management counseling in children [5]. Since lifestyle change is vitally important in childhood obesity, particularly to support the child and the family that the child lives with, these issues will be largely the focus of this chapter. These lifestyle changes include nutrition, physical activity, sleep, and other habits to help achieve healthy child growth. There are a range of treatment options available including pharmacotherapy and surgery which may be added to lifestyle changes in those children who have severe obesity and comorbid conditions.

DOI: 10.1201/9781003099116-11

10.2   KEY RESOURCES

A number of documents can help clinicians who wish to become more knowledge-able about treating childhood obesity. These include the following:

- Expert Committee Recommendations 2007 for Primary Care Practice [6]
- 2013 Scientific Statement on Severe Obesity in Children and Adolescents from the American Heart Association [7]
- 2017 Endocrine Society Clinical Practice Guidelines for Pediatric Obesity [8]
- United States Preventive Service Task Force (USPSTF) Statement on Screening for Obesity in Children and Adolescents [9]

10.3   DEFINITION

Obesity refers to excess adiposity. The accepted clinical measure in both children and adults is body mass index (BMI) which is weight in kilograms divided by height in meters^2 [10]. For children over the age of two, it is important to use the CDC BMI Growth Chart for Children 2–20 [11], which utilizes the following definition:

- Overweight (BMI $\geq$ 85th percentile – 94th percentile for age and sex)
- Obese (BMI $\geq$ 95th percentile for age and sex)
- Severely obese (BMI $\geq$ 120% of percentile for age and sex or $\geq$35 kg/m^2, whichever is lower) [7]
- For children less than the age of two, utilize WHO Weight for Length Growth Chart for 1–24 months. These charts define overweight as weight for recumbent length or age and sex $\geq$ 97.7 percentile [8].

10.4   ETIOLOGIES

As in adults, childhood obesity results from complex interactions between lifestyle, genetics, epigenetics, biopsychological, and socioeconomic social environmental factors [12]. Major etiologies are presented in Table 10.1.

10.5   COMORBID CONDITIONS

The effects of a given degree of obesity in children on various body systems may differ from the effects seen in adults. Obesity may worsen respiratory symptoms in children due to the smaller airway diameter [13]. Some orthopedic problems such as Blount Disease or Slipped Carpal Tunnel Femoral Epiphysis (SCFE) can occur prior to fusion of growth plates. Virtually every organ system can have adverse effects from childhood obesity including cardiovascular disease (CVD) [14,15], where childhood obesity increases the risk of coronary heart disease; endocrine, where childhood obesity increases the risk of type 2 diabetes (T2DM) [16–18]; and gastrointestinal, where nonalcoholic fatty liver disease may be increased in child-hood obesity.

TABLE 10.1
Etiologies of Childhood Obesity

	Key Clinical Features	Examples
Lifestyle	Normal linear growth Generalized distribution of excess adiposity	Socioenvironmental and personal factors influencing nutrition, physical activity, sedentary behaviors, and energy balance including: • Access to healthy foods • Daily screen time • Sleep quantity
Endocrinologic	Decreased linear growth	• Hypothyroidism (untreated) • Cushing Syndrome
Hypothalamic Dysfunction	Pituitary hormone deficiencies Increased hunger/poor satiety	• Treatment of hypothalamic/pituitary tumors (e.g. surgery/radiation for craniopharyngioma) • Direct effects of a tumor, trauma, or inflammatory disease
Medications	Weight gain temporally associated with medication initiation	• Atypical antipsychotics, systemic corticosteroids, and some mood stabilizers, antidepressants, and anticonvulsants
Genetic syndromes[14]	Severe obesity before age 5, developmental delay, dysmorphic features, and/or hyperphagia	Developmental delay + dysmorphic features • Prader-Willi syndrome • Bardet-Biedl syndrome • Albright hereditary osteodystrophy • (+) Hyperphagia without developmental delay or dysmorphic features • MC4R[a] deficiency • Leptin/leptin receptor deficiency • POMC[b] deficiency

[a] MC4R (Melanocortin 4 receptor).
[b] POMC (Proopiomelanocortin).
Moore J, Haemer M, Childhood Obesity In Rippe JM, *Lifestyle Medicine*, 3rd edition. CRC Press (Boca Raton) 2019. Used with permission of the Editor Dr. James Rippe.

10.6   PREVENTION OF CHILDHOOD OBESITY

• *Risk and protective factors*: Risk factors for the development of child-hood obesity have now been demonstrated in a number of studies to arise in the preconception and prenatal stages of life [19]. Postnatally, risk fac-tors associated with childhood obesity include sugar-sweetened beverage intake, increased screen time, decreased sleep duration, early adiposity rebound (to the point where BMI begins to increase from its natal to early childhood), and prior adverse family functioning, which includes violence or abuse [20,21]. Protective factors include increased physical activity, increased family, and school and/or community involvement in prevention efforts. All of these represent possible targets for intervention. Evidence of the association between breastfeeding and prevention of childhood obesity is mixed [22]. However, it should be noted that exclusive breastfeeding is recommended for the first 6 months of life for a variety of reasons [23].

- *Screening*: Early recognition of weight gain paired with early intervention strategies may prevent progression to overweight or obesity. The American Academy of Pediatrics recommends that all children should be screened in primary care at least annually for excess weight using age and sex-specific BMI percentiles for children over the age of two or weight for length percentiles for children under the age of two.
- *Effectiveness of prevention interventions*: Strong evidence exists to support the interventions already listed as generating meaningful reductions in BMI [24]. A meta-analysis of obesity prevention programs demonstrated the strongest evidence for obesity prevention came from the combined diet – physical activity interventions delivered in school with both home and community components. These results underscore the importance of a collaborative approach to prevent childhood obesity.

10.7   TREATMENT OF CHILDHOOD OBESITY

- *Overview of treatment goals*: The weight management treatment plan should adopt an overall holistic view of the child and family and should include improving quality of life, family functioning, healthy child development, and meaningful BMI change that will yield physical and mental health benefits. Families should be encouraged to participate in shared decision-making with an emphasis on their values, cultural beliefs, and socioeconomic challenges.
- *Clinical weight loss goals*: Weight loss goals need to be flexible and guided by the child's age, degree of excess weight at baseline, presence of comorbidities, and the patient/family's readiness to change. A good endpoint is a BMI less than the 95th percentile which is essential to reverse cardiometabolic risk. In some children, a BMI less than 85th percentile is advisable [25]. There are important differences in the relationship between BMI and body adiposity in different racial/ethnic groups which should guide the degree of weight loss for each individual child. Recommended rate of weight loss should also be geared by age [6]. For example, 2- to 5 year olds goals might be weight maintenance or up to one pound/month, while 6- to 11 year olds goals might be loss of one pound/month to two pounds/month, and 12- to 18 year olds one to two pounds/week. If more rapid weight losses occur, an investigation on healthy weight loss behaviors and methods should be undertaken. An excellent way of thinking about weight loss and metabolism is the NIH Body Weight Planner which accounts for decreased metabolism after weight loss [26].
- *Interpreting treatment effects* – Outcome measures reported in childhood obesity studies have lacked standardization which makes it difficult to compare conclusions. The most widely reported measure is change in BMI Z-Score. However, it should be noted that the BMI Z-score is not valid for children or adolescents with severe obesity [27]. BMI growth charts can facilitate the monitoring of weight trends in severely obese patients.

- *2007 Expert Committee Staged Intervention Framework*: – The 2007 Expert Committee Guidelines propose a structure for healthcare delivery of pediatric obesity interventions. This was divided into four stages which provided increasingly intensive interventions, beginning with structured weight management in the primary care setting all the way to comprehensive, multidisciplinary management in a tertiary care center [6]. Movement through these stages is dependent upon the severity of the patient's obesity, comorbidities, age, family motivation to change, available resources, and progress in treatment. The primary goal of treatment is permanent healthy lifestyle habits. A variety of models that implement a treatment based on this framework are in the following sections.
- *Behaviorally based multicomponent lifestyle treatment*:
  - *Overview*: Behaviorally based lifestyle interventions are recommended as the first line of treatment for childhood obesity. Most of these interventions target more than one behavior such as nutrition, physical activity, and sleep and are typically referred to as "multimodal" or "multicomponent" interventions [6–8]. A Cochran review of these interventions demonstrated positive effects on weight status.
  - *Family-based behavioral treatment (FBT)*: This intervention is the most extensively tested behavioral pediatric weight management technique which involves treating both the child and the parents. FBT is typically delivered in 16 weekly sessions and involves nutrition (using the traffic light diet paradigm), behavior (e.g. self-monitoring), and physical activity [28,29]. FBT has been demonstrated to have a positive impact on weight. However, the lack of insurance coverage and lack of sufficient training have been barriers to widespread adoption.
  - *Mind, exercise, nutrition...Do it (MEND)*: MEND is one of the most commonly implemented, community delivered, family-centered, multicomponent, pediatric weight management intervention [30]. It was developed in England in 2004, and in the United States, it is often delivered through partnership with local YMCAs.
- *Office-based interventions*: One type of office-based intervention involves motivational interviewing (MI) [31]. This has been demonstrated to be an effective personal, evidence-based tool and has the advantage of being able to be utilized either in a one-on-one setting or in group settings. (See also Chapter 7.) The American Academy of Pediatrics "Change Talk: Childhood Obesity" is a free, online source that can help providers develop MI skills [32].
- *Nutritional interventions*
  - *Balanced hypocaloric reduction*: This is often a first-line treatment and involves a balanced reduction in calories. These are typically accomplished through individualized, small changes and are matched to the family's readiness to change. This approach can be utilized in a variety of practice settings [6,8].
  - *Traffic light diet*: The traffic light diet is often used to help achieve balance in moderate to high caloric diet restriction. It is the core nutrition

component of multidisciplinary FBT programs. The system basically divides foods into green (low calorie, no limit), yellow (intermediate calorie eaten in moderation), and red (high calorie and all sugar-sweetened beverages, avoid). Families are instructed to limit red foods to less than five/week [32].

- *Ideal macronutrient composition*: There is not one specific dietary macronutrient composition that is clearly superior to achieving significant and sustained improvements in BMI. As in adults, there is some evidence that a low carb, high protein diet may be superior in the short term but, as in adults, there are no long-term data to suggest that this is superior to other macronutrient-based diets [33].
- *Very low-calorie diets (VLCD)*: VLCDs typically provide 500–800 kcal/day. These are delivered as high protein, low carb, low fat, micronutrient enhanced liquids. There are some data that suggest that these may work in the short term for individuals with high levels of obesity but these, along with other meal replacement diets, are not very well studied either in children or adolescents [34].
- *Meal replacement products*: Meal replacement products have not been shown to result in superior sustained weight loss compared to isocaloric diets with conventional foods in adolescents.
- *Physical activity and sedentary behavior interventions. (See also Chapter 5)*:
  - *Physical activity*: Physical activity is an important adjunct to nutritional and behavioral lifestyle interventions to achieve small reductions in weight outcomes at very low risk [35–37]. The power of regular physical activity in children has been amply documented in the Physical Activity Guidelines for American 2018 (PAGA) Scientific Report [38]. As with adults, the independent effect of physical activity on weight loss is less clear, but there are multiple other benefits of physical activity in children, both with obesity and at healthy weight. These include improvements in cardiorespiratory fitness, vascular function, and reduction in cardiometabolic risk factors. The PAGA 2018 recommends that children 6–17 years of age engage in at least 60 minutes/day of moderate to vigorous physical activity with a combination of aerobic (e.g. fast walking, biking), muscle strengthening (e.g. playing on a jungle gym, resistance exercise), and bone strengthening (e.g. jumping rope, activities). For children 5 years of age or under the recommendation from the PAGA 2018 is for at least 60 minutes/day of unstructured physical activity, plus daily structured physical activity for 30 minutes (1–3 year olds) and 60 minutes (3–5 year olds). Children should also engage in less sedentary time. Physical activity in children with obesity may also bring improvement in children's body image and motivation and desire to lead a physically active lifestyle [39].
  - *Sedentary behavior*: As documented in PAGA 2018, sedentary behavior is an independent risk factor for multiple metabolic conditions, including obesity. In children 5–17 years old, sedentary behavior is associated

with higher cardiometabolic risk, lower fitness, and lower self-esteem. Screen time is particularly prevalent in children [40]. In 2016, media use policy from the American Academy of Pediatrics (AA) recommends the following: [41,42]

- *Less than* 18 *months*: no screen media, except for limited video chatting.
- 18–24 *months old*: evidence-based educational shows/apps with parent interaction.
- 2–5 *years old*: ≤1 hour of high-quality programming with an adult to promote learning.
- 5–18 *years old*: no specific maximum, but parents are encouraged to place limits to ensure adequate sleep and physical activity goals are reached, as well as creating media-free family time.
- For all age groups screens should not be accessed while eating or the hour before bedtime and no screen devices should be kept in the bedroom.

The AAP Family Media Use Digital Planning Tool can help families design individualized plans [43].

- *Sleep interventions*: Sleep is a relatively new target for pediatric obesity intervention. Data support that restricted sleep is associated with double the odds of developing obesity in childhood. With each 1 hour increase in sleep per night, there is a 0.05 kg/m^2 reduction in the early BMI gain. The National Sleep Foundation recommends the following hours of sleep per night per age: 1–2 year olds (11–14 hours), 3–5 year olds (10–13 hours), 6–13 year olds (9–11 hours), and 14–17 year olds (8–10 hours) [44]. There are some data to suggest an association between sleep restriction and unhealthy dietary patterns in children.
- *Anti-obesity medications*: In addition to ongoing intensive lifestyle efforts, in some instances anti-obesity medications may be indicated in a subset of youth with obesity [6,7]. In 2019, opinion statements from the AAP provided a framework and practical consideration for youths of anti-obesity medicine in adolescents with obesity. Pharmacotherapy for children and adolescents with obesity should be considered only after participation in an intensive lifestyle program for 6–12 months which has been unsuccessful in either curbing weight gain or improving obesity comorbidities. Weight loss medications should be administered and monitored by a clinician with experience in their use and potential adverse effects. The only FDA-approved anti-obesity medication in pediatrics is the lipase inhibitor, Orlistat (for patients ≥12 years of age) [45]. The overall effect of other potential medicines on weight is small- and long-term effects have not been studied.
- *Bariatric surgery*: Severe obesity in the United States affects approximately 8.5% of 12–19 year olds and is associated with significant cardiometabolic risk, including premature death [7]. Since there are few effective treatment options for this population bariatric surgery may be considered as a tool to achieve

significant sustained weight loss when paired with ongoing lifestyle interventions. The Teen-Longitudinal Assessment of Bariatric Surgery (Teen-LABS) which was a large multicenter, prospective trial of adolescents who underwent bariatric surgery, showed a significant reduction in weight of 27% at 3 years and a majority of patients experienced remission of T2DM, elevated blood pressure, dyslipidemia, and abnormal kidney function. Lifestyle interventions play a critical role in both the preoperative period and lifelong after surgery [46].

10.8 SUMMARY/CONCLUSIONS

Pediatric obesity has grown dramatically in prevalence over the past three decades. The prevalence of obesity amongst 2–19 year olds in the United States is 18.5%. Clinicians who are treating children with obesity should become skilled in all aspects of this difficult condition. A variety of tools are available through the American Academy of Pediatrics to assist in this process.

CLINICAL APPLICATIONS

- Use motivational interviewing and other behavior change techniques to help families select and achieve attainable lifestyle change goals.
- When available, contact families to intensive, multidisciplinary family centers interventions (optimally ≥26 contact hours/year).

REFERENCES

1. Ogden C., Carroll M., Lawman H., et al. Trends in obesity prevalence among children and adolescents in the United States, 1988–1994 through 2013–2014. *JAMA*. 2016;315:2292–9.
2. Ogden C., Carroll M., Kit B., et al. Prevalence of childhood and adult obesity in the United States, 2011–2012. *JAMA*. 2014;311:806.
3. Skinner A., Skelton J. Prevalence and trends in obesity and severe obesity among children in the United States, 1999–2012. *JAMA Pediatr*. 2014;168:561.
4. Vine M., Hargreaves M., Briefel R., et al. Expanding the role of primary care in the prevention and treatment of childhood obesity: A review of clinic- and community-based recommendations and interventions. *J Obes*. 2013;2013:1–17.
5. Klein J., Sesselberg T., Johnson M., et al. Adoption of body mass index guidelines for screening and counseling in pediatric practice. *Pediatrics*. 2010;125:265–72.
6. Barlow S., Expert Committee. Expert committee recommendations regarding the prevention, assessment, and treatment of child and adolescent overweight and obesity: Summary report. *Pediatrics*. 2007;120(Suppl 4):S164–192.
7. Kelly A., Barlow S., Rao G., et al. Severe obesity in children and adolescents: Identification, associated health risks, and treatment approaches: A scientific statement from the American Heart Association. *Circulation*. 2013;128:1689–712.
8. Styne D., Arslanian S., Connor E., et al. Pediatric obesity-assessment, treatment, and prevention: An endocrine society clinical practice guideline. *J Clin Endocrinol Metab*. 2017;102:709–57.
9. US Preventive Services Task Force, Grossman D., Bibbins-Domingo K., Curry S., et al. Screening for obesity in children and adolescents: US preventive services task force recommendation statement. *JAMA*. 2017;317:2417.

10. Freedman D., Sherry B. The validity of BMI as an indicator of body fatness and risk among children. *Pediatrics.* 2009;124(Suppl 1):S23–34.
11. Center for Disease Control and Prevention National Center for Health Statistics. Clinical Growth Charts Children 2 to 20 years 2000.
12. van Dijk S., Molloy P., Varinli H., et al. Members of EpiSCOPE. Epigenetics and human obesity. *Int J Obes.* 2005;2015(39):85–97.
13. Joosten K., Larramona H., Miano S., et al. How do we recognize the child with OSAS? OSAS diagnoses in children. *Pediatr Pulmonol.* 2017;52:260–71.
14. Expert Panel on Integrated Guidelines for Cardiovascular Health and Risk Reduction in Children and Adolescents. Expert panel on integrated guidelines for cardiovascular health and risk reduction in children and adolescents: Summary report. *Pediatrics.* 2011;128:S213–56.
15. Flynn J., Kaelber D., Baker-Smith C., et al. Clinical practice guideline for screening and management of high blood pressure in children and adolescents. *Pediatrics.* 2017;140:e20171904.
16. Haemer M., Grow H., Fernandez C., et al. Addressing prediabetes in childhood obesity treatment programs: Support from research and current practice. *Child Obes.* 2014;10:292–303.
17. Kelsey M., Zeitler P. Insulin resistance of puberty. *Curr Diab Rep.* 2016;16:64.
18. Mayer-Davis E., Lawrence J., Dabelea D., et al. Incidence trends of type 1 and type 2 diabetes among youths, 2002–2012. *N Engl J Med.* 2017;376:1419–29.
19. Kaar J., Crume T., Brinton J., et al. Maternal obesity, gestational weight gain, and offspring adiposity: The exploring perinatal outcomes among children study. *J Pediatr.* 2014;165:509–15.
20. Hughes A., Sherriff A., Ness A., et al. Timing of adiposity rebound and adiposity in adolescence. *Pediatrics.* 2014;134:e1354–1361.
21. Ip E., Marshall S., Saldana S., et al. Determinants of adiposity rebound timing in children. *J Pediatr.* 2017;184:151–156.e2.
22. Yan J., Liu L., Zhu Y., et al. The association between breastfeeding and childhood obesity: a meta-analysis. *BMC Pub Health.* 2014;14:1267.
23. Section on Breastfeeding. Breastfeeding and the use of human milk. *Pediatrics.* 2012;129:e827–841.
24. Waters E., de Silva-Sanigorski A., Burford B., et al. Interventions for preventing obesity in children. In: The Cochrane Collaboration, editor. *Cochrane Database of Systematic Reviews*, Chichester, UK: John Wiley & Sons, Ltd, 2011.
25. Juonala M., Magnussen C., Berenson G., et al. Childhood adiposity, adult adiposity, and cardiovascular risk factors. *N Engl J Med.* 2011;365:1876–85.
26. National Institute of Diabetes and Digestive and Kidney Diseases. Body Weight Planner 2018.
27. Freedman D., Butte N., Taveras E., et al. BMI z-Scores are a poor indicator of adiposity among 2- to 19-year-olds with very high BMIs, NHANES 1999–2000 to 2013–2014. *Obes Silver Spring Md.* 2017;25:739–46.
28. Epstein L., Wing R., Steranchak L., et al. Comparison of family-based behavior modification and nutrition education for childhood obesity. *J Pediatr Psychol* 1980;5:25–36.
29. Wilfley D., Saelens B., Stein R., et al. Dose, content, and mediators of family-based treatment for childhood obesity: A multisite randomized clinical trial. *JAMA Pediatr.* 2017;171:1151–9.
30. Mind, Exercise, Nutrition...Do It! (MEND) 2018.
31. Resnicow K., Harris D., Wasserman R., et al. Advances in motivational interviewing for pediatric obesity: Results of the brief motivational interviewing to reduce body mass index trial and future directions. *Pediatr Clin North Am.* 2016;63:539–62.

32. Epstein L., Wing R., Koeske R., et al. Child and parent weight loss in family-based behavior modification programs. *J Consult Clin Psychol.* 1981;49:674–85.

33. Gow M.L., Ho M., Burrows T., et al. Impact of dietary macronutrient distribution on BMI and cardiometabolic outcomes in overweight and obese children and adolescents: A systematic review. *Nutr Rev.* 2014;72:453–70.

34. Brown M., Klish W., Hollander J., et al. A high protein, low calorie liquid diet in the treatment of very obese adolescents: Long-term effect on lean body mass. *Am J Clin Nutr.* 1983;38:20–31.

35. Colquitt J., Loveman E., O'Malley C., et al. Diet, physical activity, and behavioural interventions for the treatment of overweight or obesity in preschool children up to the age of 6 years. In: The Cochrane Collaboration, editor. *Cochrane Database of Systematic Reviews*, Chichester, UK: John Wiley & Sons, Ltd, 2016.

36. Mead E., Brown T., Rees K., et al. Diet, physical activity and behavioural interventions for the treatment of overweight or obese children from the age of 6 to 11 years. In: The Cochrane Collaboration, editor. *Cochrane Database of Systematic Reviews*, Chichester, UK: John Wiley & Sons, Ltd; 2017.

37. Al-Khudairy L., Loveman E., Colquitt J., et al. Diet, physical activity and behavioural interventions for the treatment of overweight or obese adolescents aged 12 to 17 years. *Cochrane Database Syst Rev.* 2017;6:CD012691.

38. Physical Activity Guidelines for Americans 2015–2020. n.d.

39. National Association for Sport and Physical Education. A Statement of Physical Activity Guidelines for Children from Birth to Age 5. 2nd ed. n.d.

40. Carson V., Hunter S., Kuzik N., et al. Systematic review of sedentary behaviour and health indicators in school-aged children and youth: An update. *Appl Physiol Nutr Metab Physiol Appl Nutr Metab.* 2016;41:S240–265.

41. Council on Communications and Media. Media and young minds. *Pediatrics.* 2016;138:e20162591.

42. Council on Communications and Media. Media use in school-aged children and adolescents. *Pediatrics.* 2016;138:e20162592.

43. Family Media Plan 2018.

44. Hirshkowitz M., Whiton K., Albert S., et al. National Sleep Foundation's updated sleep duration recommendations: Final report. *Sleep Health.* 2015;1:233–43.

45. James W., Caterson I., Coutinho W., et al. Effect of sibutramine on cardiovascular outcomes in overweight and obese subjects. *N Engl J Med.* 2010;363:905–17.

46. Inge T., Courcoulas A., Jenkins T., et al. Weight loss and health status 3 years after bariatric surgery in adolescents. *N Engl J Med.* 2016;374:113–23.

11 Adiposity-Based Chronic Disease
A New Diagnostic Term

James M. Rippe, MD
Rippe Lifestyle Institute
University of Massachusetts Medical School

CONTENTS

11.1 INTRODUCTION

Intracellular fat deposition plays a central role in energy metabolism. With this concept, several investigators, led by Dr. Jeffrey Mechanick, have suggested that this deposition allows for the classification of a new diagnostic term called "Adiposity-Based Chronic Disease" (ABCD) [1,2]. This classification allows for an approach both clinically and also from a research perspective [3–5]. Fat deposition occurs in a variety of body distributions including adipose tissue as well as muscle (myocytes) and liver cells (hepatocytes).

Depending on where fat is distributed, it directly or indirectly participates in energy metabolism through intermediary metabolism and hormone receptor signal

DOI: 10.1201/9781003099116-12

TABLE 11.1

Defining Characteristics of ABCD.[a]

Adiposity variable metric

Increased mass Anthropometrics (e.g. weight, BMI)

Body composition imaging

Abnormal distribution anthropometrics (e.g. WC, WHR)

Body composition imaging

Abnormal function adipokine/cytokine levels (e.g. adiponectin, leptin)

[a] ABCD is differentiated from obesity by Abbreviations: ABCD, adiposity-based chronic disease; BMI, body mass index; WC, waist circumference; WHR, waist-to-hip ratio.
    Components of adiposity-based chronic disease.

Source: Via M, Mechanick J. Adiposity-Based Chronic Disease a New Diagnostic Term. In Rippe JM: *Lifestyle Medicine*, 3rd ed., CRC Press (Boca Raton), 2019. Used with permission of the editor Dr. James Rippe.

transduction which leads to states of inflammation, insulin resistance, abnormal food-seeking behavior, and organ dysfunction.

The term ABCD refers to the chronic disease state causally associated with abnormalities of adiposity. This is depicted in Table 11.1

ABCD is distinguished from the term "obesity" which is currently defined as having a body mass index (BMI) greater than certain defined cutoffs (e.g. 30 kg/m^2 or greater for Caucasians). ABCD may be supported by anthropometric measurements such as BMI and waist circumference, body composition technologies (e.g. dual X-ray absorptiometry (DEXA), as well as other imaging studies such as computerized technology) [3,4]. Obesity may also be defined by a variety of markers including factors such as triglycerides and markers of inflammation.

A variety of conflicting health messages have emerged over many years about the definition and causes of obesity and a variety of theories about the best way to treat it. This confusion about definition and terminology has often led to health care professionals finding it difficult to implement effective therapies [6,7]. The concept of ABCD intends to emphasize the unhealthy nature of excessive adiposity beyond simple BMI or body weight and includes abnormal body fat distribution and changes in adipocyte secretome patterns.

Proponents of ABCD feel that it allows for a more focused set of behavioral as well as pharmaceutical and procedural interventions. This may lead to more widespread adoption of intensive lifestyle modification.

11.2 CONSEQUENCES OF ABCD

The health consequences of ABCD include metabolic, cardiovascular, orthopedic, gastrointestinal, psychiatric, and oncologic risk. These are categorized in Table 11.2.

While there is a considerable degree of variation, the effects of adipose tissue accumulation lead some investigators to say that it is possible to have excess adipose

TABLE 11.2
ABCD-Related Conditions[a]

Condition	Relative Risk	ABCD Component		
		Adiposity Amount	Characteristic Adipose Distribution	Abnormal Adipocyte Function
Metabolic				
Type 2 diabetes	7.7	++++	++++	++++
Polycystic ovary syndrome	1.5	+	++	++
Hepatosteatosis	1.9	++	+++	++
Obstructive sleep apnea	3.6	+++	++	++
Cardiovascular				
Hypertension	2.0	++	++	+
Atherosclerotic disease	1.6	++	++	+++
Arrhythmia	1.49	+	+++	++
Orthopedic				
Osteoarthritis	1.39	+	+	-
Tendon injuries	1.7	++	++	++
Gout	2.2	++	+	+
Gonadal Function				
Infertility (women)	1.2	+	++	++
Hypothalamic hypogonadism (men)	1.6	++	+++	+++
Gastrointestinal				
Cholelithiasis	1.8	++	+	++
Psychiatric				
Depression	2.0	++	+++	+++
Cancer				
Obesity-related (esophageal, colon, pancreatic, prostate, kidney, liver, gall bladder)	1.5	++	+	+

[a] Relative risk compared to non-obese population

Via M, Mechanick J. Adiposity-Based Chronic Disease a New Diagnostic Term. In Rippe JM: *Lifestyle Medicine*, 3rd ed., CRC Press (Boca Raton), 2019. Used with permission of the editor Dr. James Rippe.

tissue and remain "metabolically healthy" (MHO). Over time, even individuals with MHO have an increased risk of T2DM, insulin resistance, and cardiovascular disease (CVD) [8,9]. Importantly, advocates of ABCD feel that it emphasizes the importance of lifestyle choices to help ameliorate the various conditions associated with adverse amounts of adipose tissue.

11.3   INTENSIVE LIFESTYLE INTERVENTION

Intensive lifestyle intervention is appropriate for individuals with ABCD. For example, a healthy dietary pattern is recommended which will be enhanced by adherence and sustainability which can be based on behavioral assessments such as motivational interviewing (see also Chapter 7). A dietary pattern of high fruits, vegetables, nuts, carbohydrates, and controlled amounts of meats, fish, and negligible amounts of processed foods and sugar-containing beverages will provide great benefit for patients with ABCD [10]. Of course, these guidelines have been widely demonstrated to be effective in a variety of metabolic conditions including CVD and T2DM. Diets such as the Mediterranean Diet [11], the New Nordic Diet [12], the Ornish Diet [13], and the Dietary Approaches to Stop Hypertension (DASH) diet [14] are examples of diets based on these premises.

Multiple recommendations from organizations such as the American Heart Association (AHA) and the American Diabetes Association (ADA), as well as the Academy of Nutrition and Dietetics (AND), all fundamentally support the concept of healthy eating as does the Dietary Guidelines for Americans 2020–2025 [15]. These diets have been demonstrated in multiple studies to lower inflammation and help with weight control as well as lowering risk factors for various metabolic diseases.

In addition to following this type of dietary pattern, increasing the amounts of physical activity and many other lifestyle factors are important for lowering the risk factors for ABCD as well as multiple other chronic diseases. The Physical Activity Guidelines for Americans 2018 Scientific Report provides ample evidence of the multiple benefits of following a physically active lifestyle [16]. Unfortunately, only about 25% of individuals in the US achieve enough regular physical activity to lower their risk of various chronic diseases including obesity.

11.4   SLEEP HYGEINE

Sleep is an important and often underestimated component of multiple aspects of a healthy lifestyle including metabolism. Sleep affects hypothalamic function, cortisol release, thyroid function, hepatic glucose production, brown fat activation, and insulin resistance [17].

In the modern era, average sleep duration has been declining. In addition to reduced sleep time, the presence of insomnia, defined as waking in the middle of the night at least three times weekly, is reported among 25%–35% of adults.

In children, no upper limit of healthy sleep has been identified, but a longer duration of sleep is associated with reduced amounts of adiposity, improved quality of life, and improved academic success. For adults, between 7 and 9 hours of sleep is recommended nightly, while 8–10 hours of sleep is recommended for adolescents. Disordered sleep is disruptive to circadian rhythms and is associated with weight gain. Obstructive sleep apnea (OSA) is highly prevalent in adults with obesity and disruptive to healthy sleep [18,19]. In one longitudinal study, a 10% increase in body weight was associated with a six-fold increase in OSA. Thus, proper sleep hygiene is important to multiple metabolic parameters including ABCD, CVD, and T2DM.

11.5 STRESS REDUCTION

Human stress plays a significant role in a variety of metabolic abnormalities. Chronic stress is associated with multiple aspects of dysglycemia and ABCD and also associated with hypothalamic dysfunction, increased consumption of palatable and calorie-dense foods, and reduced physical activity. The hormonal profile with chronic stress includes elevations of cortisol and catecholamines, and is part of an insulin-resistant state [20,21].

Modalities to address stress and lessen pathophysiologic effects of stress may be beneficial to a variety of metabolic conditions including ABCD. Some techniques for stress reduction include relaxation response, mindfulness meditation, and mindful exercise such as Yoga. Such mindfulness techniques represent promising lifestyle interventions for multiple chronic diseases including ABCD [22,23]. Several studies have shown that mindfulness techniques in individuals with obesity improve the quality of life and lower risk for cardiovascular events and markers of inflammation. Studies related to Yoga have shown similar results.

11.6 ANTIBIOTIC USE AND THE MICROBIOME

11.6.1 ANTIBIOTIC USE BY HUMANS

Antibiotics are critical for the treatment of infectious diseases of bacterial or fungal origin. Antibiotic use can also affect microflora residing within the gastrointestinal (GI) tract [24]. Lifestyle changes that affect gut microbiota can indirectly lead to a variety of changes in chronic conditions such as ABCD. The microbes in the gut effect energy homeostasis through the metabolism of sugar and fiber present in the stool and produce short-chain fatty acids that are available for utilization by the host. Approximately 5%–10% of daily calorie consumption is obtained in this fashion. This is an area of active research since the impact of microflora may be significant for both weight gain and obesity. Although the science in this area is in its infancy, and the potential for multiple confounding factors exists, a reasonable approach would be to minimize the use of antibiotics in medical practice which may help with weight gain and influence other aspects of ABCD – particularly among infants and children.

11.6.2 ANTIBIOTIC USE IN FARMING

The use of antibiotics outside the medical field may also play an indirect role in the development of ABCD. For example, widespread use of antibiotics by livestock farmers yields animals that gain weight faster and require less feed [25]. It should be noted that changes within the livestock microbiome have also been reported. Whether this impacts the likelihood of developing ABCD is not known; however, it should be investigated in the future.

11.7 ENDOCRINE DISRUPTORS

A number of chemical compounds may affect hormone signaling. Some of these endocrine-disrupting compounds (EDC) have been demonstrated to shown to affect adipose tissue accumulation, distribution, and function. For example, childhood exposure to bisphenol A has been associated with weight gain and obesity. Many other EDCs can affect energy metabolism and could potentially contribute to ABCD [26]. This area is a subject of ongoing research.

11.8   ALCOHOL MODERATION

It is well known that excessive alcohol intake is associated with a number of adverse health outcomes. In contrast, moderate alcohol consumption, particularly wine, has been demonstrated to improve markers of insulin resistance, cholesterol levels, and systemic inflammation, suggesting improvement in adipose function [27,28]. Moderate consumption of alcohol in several studies has been shown to yield reduced insulin resistance. Of course, excessive alcohol consumption and lead to a variety of adverse consequences including motor vehicle accidents and increased risk of a variety of cardiac issues.

11.9   MOOD

Disorders of mood, such as depression and anxiety, have a relationship with weight gain and risk of ABCD. For example, obesity and depression often occur together in the same patient and may be due in part to common molecular mechanisms including altered hypothalamic-pituitary-adrenal axis signaling and increased systemic inflammation [29,30]. In addition, many anti-depressant medications increase weight gain and adiposity. These include tricyclic antidepressants, selective serotonin reuptake inhibitors, and monoamine oxidase inhibitors. Antipsychotics may also produce weight gain and insulin resistance [31]. Weight loss may reduce these issues in patients with ABCD. In addition, cognitive behavioral therapy (CBT) can improve mood disorders and weight loss. Health care professionals especially in psychiatry can implement CBT if they are properly trained. (See also Chapter 7.)

11.10   COMMUNITY ENGAGEMENT

Community engagement may reduce the likelihood and impact of ABCD. It is well known that personal contacts and community involvement can have an impact in this area. Such programs as those that engage whole families in healthy dietary patterns, physical activity, and well-being have been shown to diminish childhood obesity. (See also Chapter 10.) A significant barrier to participation in family programs is denial or lack of recognition by parents with children who are overweight or obese. The role of community engagement in driving healthy behaviors may be enhanced with the use of virtual online communities. This area is only beginning to be studied.

11.11   TRANSCULTURALZATION

The cultural background of each individual significantly impacts lifestyle choices and response to advice from clinicians. For example, some cultures traditionally place value on weight gain as a marker of wealth, higher social standing, and overall well-being [32]. The World Health Organization (WHO) and others have tended to respond to these issues around the globe. In addition, ethnic variation can be related to an increased prevalence of ABCD in certain ethnic groups. For example, in East Asian and Indian populations, a waist-to-hip ratio and BMI do not capture the full risk conferred by adiposity.

11.12   SUMMARY/CONCLUSION

Obesity has continued to grow as a worldwide pandemic. Combatting obesity is a high priority in public health around the world. Multiple lifestyle factors have been identified related to dietary patterns and physical activity. ABCD potentially incorporates not only body weight and BMI but also healthy and unhealthy fat distribution and secretory functions of body fat. This conceptualization might lead to early identification and treatment of individuals who are susceptible to these abnormalities.

CLINICAL APPLICATIONS

- Much has been learned in the past two decades about the role of adipocytes.
- The concept of adiposity-based chronic disease (ABCD) emphasizes the pathophysiology of adipocytes.
- The identification of ABCD may allow early intensive lifestyle intervention and lower the likelihood of weight gain and obesity.

REFERENCES

1. Via M., Mechanick J. Adiposity-based chronic disease a new diagnostic term. In Rippe J.M. (ed.) *Lifestyle Medicine*, 3rd ed., Boca Raton, FL: CRC Press, 2019.
2. Katsiki N., Mikhailidis D., Gotzamani-Psarrakou A., et al., Effect of various treatments on leptin, adiponectin, ghrelin and neuropeptide Y in patients with type 2 diabetes mellitus. *Expert Opin Ther Targets*. 2011;15:401–420.
3. Kouli G., Panagiotakos D., Kyrou I., et al., Visceral adiposity index and 10-year cardiovascular disease incidence: The ATTICA study. *Nutr Metab Cardiovasc Dis*. 2017;27(10):881–889.
4. Mechanick J., Zhao S., Garvey W. The adipokine-cardiovascular-lifestyle network: Translation to clinical practice. *J Am Coll Cardiol*. 2016;68:1785–1803.
5. Garvey W., Mechanick J., Brett E., et al., American association of clinical endocrinologists and American college of endocrinology comprehensive clinical practice guidelines for medical care of patients with obesity. *Endocr Pract*. 2016;22(Suppl 3):1–203.
6. Via M., Mechanick J. Obesity as a disease. *Curr Obes Rep*. 2014;3:291–297.
7. Brodesser-Akner T. Losing it in the anti-dieting age. In: *The New York Times* Aug 6, 2017 P. MM35.
8. Kim N., Seo J., Cho H., et al., Risk of the development of diabetes and cardiovascular disease in metabolically healthy obese people: The Korean genome and epidemiology study. *Medicine (Baltimore)* 2016;95:e3384.
9. Roberson L., Aneni E., Maziak W., et al., Beyond BMI: The "Metabolically healthy obese" phenotype & its association with clinical/subclinical cardiovascular disease and all-cause mortality: A systematic review. *BMC Public Health*. 2014;14:14.

10. Leung A., Chan R., Sea M., et al., An overview of factors associated with adherence to lifestyle modification programs for weight management in adults. *Int J Environ Res Pub Health.* 2017;14(8):922.
11. Estruch R., Ros E., Salas-Salvado J., et al., Primary prevention of cardiovascular disease with a Mediterranean diet. *N Engl J Med.* 2013;368:1279–1290.
12. Ornish D., Scherwitz L., Billings J.H., et al., Intensive lifestyle changes for reversal of coronary heart disease. *JAMA.* 1998;280:2001–2007.
13. Fritzen A., Lundsgaard A., Jordy A., et al., New Nordic diet-induced weight loss is accompanied by changes in metabolism and AMPK signaling in adipose tissue. *J Clin Endocrinol Metab.* 2015;100:3509–3519.
14. Obarzanek E., Sacks F., Vollmer W., et al., Effects on blood lipids of a blood pressure-lowering diet: The dietary approaches to stop hypertension (DASH) trial. *Am J Clin Nutr.* 2001;74:80–89.
15. U.S. Department of Agriculture and U.S. Department of Health and Human Services. Dietary Guidelines for Americans, 2020–2025. 9th Edition. December 2020. Available at DietaryGuidelines.gov. https://www.dietaryguidelines.gov/sites/default/files/2020-12/Dietary_Guidelines_for_Americans_2020-2025.pdf. Accessed January 19, 2021.
16. Physical Activity Guidelines for Americans 2018. Washington, DC https://health.gov/sites/default/files/2019-09/Physical_Activity_Guidelines_2nd_edition.pdf. Accessed August 26, 2020
17. Gruber R., Carrey N., Weiss S., et al., Position statement on pediatric sleep for psychiatrists. *J Can Acad Child Adolesc Psychiatry.* 2014;23:174–195.
18. Buman M., Kline C., Youngstedt S., et al., Sitting and television viewing: Novel risk factors for sleep disturbance and apnea risk? Results from the 2013 National Sleep Foundation Sleep in America Poll. *Chest.* 2015;147:728–734.
19. Feng Y., Zhang Z., Dong Z. Effects of continuous positive airway pressure therapy on glycaemic control, insulin sensitivity and body mass index in patients with obstructive sleep apnea and type 2 diabetes: A systematic review and meta-analysis. *NPJ Prim Care Respir Med.* 2015;25:15005.
20. Chao A., Jastreboff A., White M., et al., Stress, cortisol, and other appetite-related hormones: Prospective prediction of 6-month changes in food cravings and weight. *Obesity (Silver Spring).* 2017;25:713–720.
21. Donoho C., Weigensberg M., Emken B., et al., Stress and abdominal fat: Preliminary evidence of moderation by the cortisol awakening response in Hispanic peripubertal girls. *Obesity (Silver Spring).* 2011;19:946–952.
22. Godsey J. The role of mindfulness based interventions in the treatment of obesity and eating disorders: An integrative review. *Complement Ther Med.* 2013;21:430–439.
23. O'Reilly G.A., Cook L., Spruijt-Metz D., Black D.S. Mindfulness-based interventions for obesity-related eating behaviours: A literature review. *Obes Rev* 2014;15:453–461.
24. Cox L., Blaser M. Antibiotics in early life and obesity. *Nat Rev Endocrinol.* 2015;11:182–190.
25. Jukes T. Antibiotics in animal feeds. *N Engl J Med.* 1970;282:49–50.
26. Vafeiadi M., Roumeliotaki T., Myridakis A., et al., Association of early life exposure to bisphenol A with obesity and cardiometabolic traits in childhood. *Environ Res.* 2016;146:379–387.
27. Brien S., Ronksley P., Turner B., et al., Effect of alcohol consumption on biological markers associated with risk of coronary heart disease: Systematic review and meta-analysis of interventional studies. *BMJ.* 2011;342:d636.
28. Traversy G., Chaput J. Alcohol consumption and obesity: An update. *Curr Obes Rep.* 2015;4:122–130.
29. Ubani C., Zhang J. The role of adiposity in the relationship between serum leptin and severe major depressive episode. *Psychiatry Res.* 2015;228:866–870.

30. Luppino F., de Wit L., Bouvy P. et al., Overweight, obesity, and depression: A systematic review and meta-analysis of longitudinal studies. *Arch Gen Psychiatry.* 2010;67:220–229.
31. Serretti A., Mandelli L. Antidepressants and body weight: A comprehensive review and meta-analysis. *J Clin Psychiatry.* 2010. 71:1259–1272.
32. Mechanick J., Marchetti A., Apovian C., et al., Diabetes-specific nutrition algorithm: A transcultural program to optimize diabetes and prediabetes care. *Curr Diab Rep.* 2012;12:180–194.

Section II

Obesity and Specific Medical Conditions

12 Obesity and Cardiovascular Disease

James M. Rippe, MD
Rippe Lifestyle Institute
University of Massachusetts Medical School

CONTENTS

12.1 INTRODUCTION

Both overweight and obesity represent significant risk factors for cardiovascular disease (CVD) [1–10]. The AHA lists obesity as a major risk factor for CVD, both because of its association with other risk factors (e.g. diabetes, dyslipidemias, elevated blood pressure, metabolic syndrome), but also because it serves as an independent risk factor.

The distribution of body fat also carries additional risks. Abdominal obesity is an independent risk factor for coronary heart disease (CHD) [11]. This is basically because the accumulation of intraabdominal fat produces insulin resistance which can contribute to glucose intolerance, elevated triglycerides, and low HDL as well as hypertension.

Recent estimates indicate that the prevalence of overweight (body mass index [BMI] 25–30 kg/m^2 in the United States for adult women is 30% and for adult men is approximately 40%). Estimates of obesity (BMI $\geq$ 30 kg/m^2) are currently 40% for women and approximately 35% for men. Within the obesity category, severe obesity (BMI $\geq$ 35 kg/m^2) is approximately 16% [12]. These high prevalence figures constitute a significant public health concern because of the relationship of excess body fat to multiple chronic diseases, in general, and CVD, in particular.

New guidelines were published in 2013 by the AHA and ACC and The Obesity Society (TOS) to help physicians manage obesity more effectively [13]. These guidelines make five major recommendations including the following:

- Use BMI as a first step in establishing criteria to judge potential health risks.
- Counsel patients that lifestyle changes can produce modest and sustained weight loss and achieve meaningful health benefits, while greater weight loss produces greater benefits.
- Multiple dietary therapy approaches to weight loss are acceptable for weight loss. However, the diet should be prescribed to achieve reduced caloric intake.
- Patients who are overweight or obese should be enrolled in comprehensive lifestyle interventions for weight loss delivered in programs of 6 months or longer.
- Advice should be provided to patients who might be contemplating bariatric surgery (BMI $\geq$ 40 kg/m^2) or BMI $\geq$ 30 kg/m^2 with obesity-related comorbid conditions).

It is important to recognize that the key therapeutic modalities to treat weight gain and obesity are lifestyle based, namely, increased physical activity and sound nutrition. The large National Institutes of Health Look AHEAD (Action for Health and Diabetes) Trial showed that individuals who lost 7% of body weight significantly lowered all cardiovascular risk factors, except for LDL cholesterol levels [14]. However, the rate of cardiovascular events was not reduced during the trial.

12.2   HEMODYNAMICS OF ADIPOSE TISSUE

It used to be thought that adipose tissue was largely for storage purposes in the human body. However, research over the past two decades has shown that adipocytes, particularly in the abdominal region, are highly metabolically active and supplied by an extensive capillary network. While resting blood flow in adipose tissue is considerably less than skeletal muscle, it can increase dramatically after a meal. The resting blood flow in adipose tissue is usually on the order of 2–3 ml/minute/100 g but may increase up to tenfold after a meal [15,16]. In addition to hemodynamic issues, adipose tissue represents a complex endocrine organ that excretes a variety of compounds into the bloodstream which can interact with the cardiovascular system. For example, adipose tissue is a significant source of leptin, adiponectin, insulin-like growth factor-1 (IGF-1), tumor necrosis factor alpha (TNFα), plasminogen activating factor inhibitor-1, lipoprotein lipase N circulating concentrations, and interlukin-6 (IL-6) [17–22]. It has been estimated that approximately 30% of the circulating concentrations of IL-6 originate in adipose tissue [23]. This is important since IL-6 is involved in the modulation of CRP production in the liver, and CRP appears to be a marker of chronic inflammation that can trigger acute coronary syndromes.

12.3 HEMODYNAMIC EFFECTS OF OBESITY

Obesity resembles high output or volume overload to the cardiovascular system. Left ventricular filling pressures and volume are higher in individuals who are obese than in lean individuals [24]. Total blood volume and cardiac output are also increased, thereby generating increased cardiac output [25]. The combination of higher loading pressures and the increased cardiac output may result in left ventricular dilatation and, ultimately, congestive heart failure. Left atrial enlargement may also occur. This is thought to be a result of left ventricular diastolic dysfunction. Atrial enlargement may also contribute to excess risk of atrial fibrillation observed in obese individuals [26]. Left ventricular hypertrophy is common in longstanding obesity and may result in systemic volume overload and hypertension [27]. Many of these hemodynamic issues can be partially ameliorated by weight loss.

12.4 EFFECTS ON LEFT VENTRICULAR FUNCTION

Long-standing obesity is associated with an increased risk of left ventricular systolic dysfunction and impairment of the left ventricular diastolic function [28]. Fatty infiltration of the cardiac muscle can further compound these problems and exacerbate both left ventricular systolic and diastolic dysfunction.

12.5 OBESITY AND CORONARY HEART DISEASE

Numerous studies have demonstrated that obesity correlates with established risk factors for CHD as well as constituting an independent risk. Specifically, there are well-established relationships between obesity, type 2 diabetes (T2DM), hypertension, and dyslipidemias (particularly elevated triglycerides and diminished HDL) [29]. Figure 12.1 shows the relative risk of all of these relationships increases as body mass index increases.

In addition to its association with increased risk factors for CHD, obesity also has an independent relationship with increased risk of CHD. This relationship appears to be linear over a wide range of BMI values suggesting that individuals, even at average weight at midlife, are at increased risk for CHD compared to leaner individuals. There is also an increased risk of CHD associated with increased abdominal fat which appears to be based on adverse metabolic consequences due to the highly lipolytic adipocytes in the abdominal region.

- *Pathogenesis of atherosclerosis*: A number of studies have shown that the atherosclerotic process can be manifested in children as early as 5–10 years old, since deposits of cholesterol and macrophage foam cells are present in large arteries (fatty streaks) [30,31]. This, in turn, may result in endothelial cell dysfunction and inflammation of the vessel wall. Some research

Figure 1.

Relative risks for hypertension, coronary heart disease (CHD), ischemic stroke, pulmonary embolism, and type 2 diabetes, according to body mass index up to 32 kg/m^2, after 14–16 years of follow-up, among women in the Nurses' Health Study. Relative risks for type 2 diabetes are age adjusted. Relative risks for other conditions are adjusted for age, smoking status, menopausal status, postmenopausal hormone use, parental history of myocardial infarction, oral contraceptive use (for the outcomes of hypertension, ischemic stroke, and pulmonary embolism), and parity (for the outcomes of hypertension and pulmonary embolism).

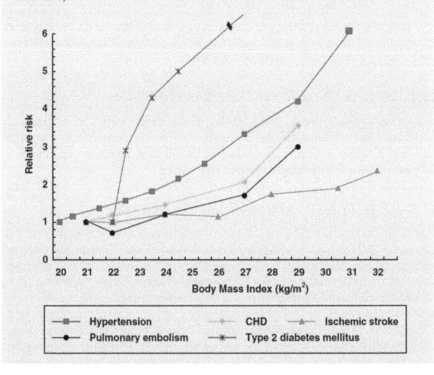

FIGURE 12.1   Risk factors for coronary heart disease based on body mass index. (Adapted from: Bassuk SS, Manson JE. Lifestyle and risk of cardiovascular disease and type 2 diabetes in women: A review of the epidemiologic evidence. *Amer J Life Med*. 2008;2:191–213.)

suggests that the risk of CHD could potentially be identified in childhood by measurement of carotid intima media thickness (IMT). With age, atherosclerotic lesions become more complex. In one study of individuals 15–30 years old who died from suicide, homicides, or accidental injury, both fatty streaks and more advanced lesions were found in the right coronary artery and were associated with obesity.

12.6   OBESITY AND RISK FACTORS FOR CORONARY HEART DISEASE

- *Obesity and hypertension*: Observational studies have consistently demonstrated a direct association between weight and blood pressure. The prevalence of hypertension is increased between two and fourfold in individuals who are obese [32,33]. It has been estimated that more than one-third of cases of hypertension in the United States are associated with obesity. In addition, weight gain is associated with an increased risk of developing hypertension. A 20-pound weight gain is associated with 3 mm/Hg higher systolic and 2.3 mm/Hg higher diastolic blood pressure which results in an estimated 12% increased risk of CHD and 24% increased risk in stroke.

  A variety of mechanisms have been postulated to explain the link between obesity and hypertension [34]. Both elevated cardiac output and increased vascular resistance are observed in individuals who are obese. In addition, insulin resistance and hyperinsulinemia also frequently accompany obesity which may further contribute to an increase in the risk of hypertension in the patients who are obese.

- *Obesity and diabetes/glucose intolerance*: Bodyweight correlates strongly with both glucose intolerance and T2DM [35,36]. Not all individuals with obesity are diabetic. However, most type 2 diabetics are individuals who are obese. The link between obesity and T2DM appears to be mediated by resultant hyperinsulinemia which frequently accompanies obesity. In the Nurses' Health Trial, the risk of developing T2DM over 16 years of observation was nearly forty-fold higher in women if the amount was $\geq$35 kg/m^2 and twenty-fold higher in women with a BMI of 30–34.9 compared to women whose BMI was $\leq$23 kg/m^2. Both the U.S. Male Health Professional Follow-up Study and NHANES have revealed similar trends in males.

  Weight gain during adult years has also been associated with an increased risk of diabetes. The increase in the prevalence of developing diabetes varies from study to study with a four to twelve-fold increase in individuals who gain between 5 and 20 kg during adult years. Since over 75% of individuals with T2DM die of CHD, the links between diabetes and obesity are particularly worrisome due to the increased risk of developing CHD.

- *Obesity and dyslipidemias*: Multiple different lipid abnormalities are associated with obesity [37,38]. Higher triglyceride levels and lower HDL cholesterol are related to BMI in both men and women in all age groups. In addition, total cholesterol and LDL cholesterol in both men and women between the ages of 20–40 correlate with BMI. The etiology of these dyslipidemias is complex but may be a result of the lipolytic nature of the adipocytes, particularly in the abdominal area which results in a higher level of free fatty acids which are released into the portal circulation and contributes to a wide range of metabolic derangements and hepatic dysfunction leading to a variety of dyslipidemias.

- *Obesity and metabolic syndrome*: The prevalence of metabolic syndrome (MetS) has increased dramatically in the United States in the past 30 years.

It is now estimated that between 36% and 38% of the adults in the United States have MetS. This is a clustering of dyslipidemias (specifically elevated triglycerides and depressed HDL), glucose intolerance, hypertension, and abdominal obesity. MetS represents a significant risk factor for both diabetes and CHD. The NCEP-ATP III Guidelines recommend that individuals with metabolic syndrome be treated as though they already have CHD.

- *Obesity and vascular disease*: A variety of vascular diseases and/or conditions are frequently present in obesity. Pedal edema is common in obesity and may be related to elevated left and right ventricular filling pressures [39]. Venous thromboembolism is more common in obese individuals than in normal weight individuals and this may contribute to an increased risk of pulmonary embolism in women with obesity [40].
- *Arrhythmias*: Individuals who are obese are at increased risk for arrhythmias and sudden cardiac death [41]. Framingham data suggest that cardiac death risks in men and women with obesity can be as much as 40 times higher than the non-obese population. A prolonged QTc interval is found in approximately 30% of individuals with glucose intolerance or obesity. A prolonged QTc interval has been associated with a variety of cardiac arrhythmias. In addition, alterations in the autonomic nervous system such as increased sympathetic tone resulting in an increased heart rate have also been associated with higher increased body weight.
- *Inflammation*: There is a strong correlation between obesity and markers in inflammation including IL-6 and CRP [42]. Obesity has been likened to total body low-grade systematic inflammation. The inflammatory process may, in turn, play a role in multiple cardiac issues including endothelial dysfunction and hypertension.
- *Sleep apnea*: A variety of respiratory complications may be present in individuals with obesity [43]. Most prominent among these conditions is sleep apnea. This may be the result of respiratory insufficiency, particularly in the supine state. It has been estimated that 40 million individuals have sleep disorders. The prevalence of these disorders increases substantially in individuals with obesity. Sleep apnea can result in hypertension, and it is also associated with increased levels of CRP. Pulmonary hypertension may also accompany sleep apnea.

12.7 THE EFFECTS OF OBESITY TREATMENT ON RISK FACTORS FOR CORONARY HEART DISEASE

- *Effects of weight loss on hypertension*: Weight loss has been repeatedly demonstrated to lower both systolic and diastolic blood pressure independent of other lifestyle factors [44–46]. The National High Blood Pressure Education Program Working Group on Primary Prevention of Hypertension and the Joint National Commission on Prevention, Detection, Evaluation and Treatment of High Blood Pressure (JNC VIII) have both recommended weight loss as a primary therapeutic modality for individuals with obesity with high blood pressure [47]. Large, randomized controlled trials of weight reduction utilizing lifestyle measures in adults with high or normal blood pressure have consistently shown weight loss as the most effective lifestyle modality for lowering blood pressure in overweight or obesity.

Reduction in systolic and diastolic blood pressure on the order of 0.5–1 mm/Hg for every kg of weight loss has been repeatedly demonstrated. These reductions in blood pressure are comparable to results from many antihypertension agents. Weight loss may also serve as an adjunctive therapy to improve blood pressure control. The exact mechanism for blood pressure reduction in individuals with obesity and hypertension is not fully understood. Some mechanisms have been possibly implicated such as decreased vascular tone, increased adrenergic tone, and decreased blood volume.

- *Effects of weight loss on type 2 diabetes (T2DM) and glucose intolerance*: Intervention trials in individuals with T2DM and glucose intolerance have repeatedly shown that intentional weight loss in individuals with obesity, either alone or combined with physical activity, improves both glucose levels and insulin responsiveness [48–50]. The United States Diabetes Prevention Program (DPP) which enrolled 3,334 men and women between the ages of 25–85 years old with baseline impaired glucose intolerance (IGT) demonstrated a 58% reduction in the progression of IGT to diabetes in the lifestyle intervention group [49]. These individuals lost 5%–7% of their body weight and exercised an average of 30 minutes/day. The Finish Diabetes Prevention Study showed similar findings. The Swedish Obese Subject Study (SOS) followed obese individuals over a 10 year period without diabetes at baseline who achieved weight loss through bariatric surgery. These individuals decreased their risk of developing diabetes by 75% when compared to matched obese controls. A large, randomized control study, the Look AHEAD (Action for Health and Diabetes) Trial also showed decreased risk factors for diabetes in individuals who lost 5%–7% of their body weight.

- *Effects of weight loss on dyslipidemia*: Weight loss has been shown to result in a variety of beneficial effects on lipid profiles. It should be noted that these benefits may be somewhat confounded by nutritional components of lipid management. A meta-analysis of 70 trials utilizing diet alone showed that weight loss resulted in significant decreases in total cholesterol, triglycerides, and LDL cholesterol in individuals with dyslipidemia [51]. Significant improvements in HDL cholesterol were also achieved once individuals achieved reduced stabilized weight. Results of weight loss on lipids are less consistent than in hypertension. However, several studies have suggested that a lipid profile can result in meaningful improvements with weight loss of less than 10%. Clinically relevant changes in cholesterol/HDL ratio can occur with weight loss of 5%–10% of initial body weight.

- *Cardiopulmonary benefits of weight loss*: In addition to the reduction of risk factors for CHD, intentional weight loss can improve aspects of the physiology of the cardiovascular system in obese individuals. These include potential benefits in improvement of left ventricular systolic and diastolic function, reduction of abnormalities of high output (decreased blood volume, decreased stroke volume and decreased cardiac output, decreased left ventricular mass, and decreased filling pressures in the right and left side of the heart) [52]. In addition, improvement or no change in systemic arterial resistance, decreased resting oxygen consumption, decreased heart rate and shortened QTc intervals, and increased heart rate variability. All of these factors can contribute to improved cardiovascular hemodynamics.

- *Risks of weight loss*: While multiple benefits typically accompany weight loss in individuals with obesity, certain weight loss modalities may result in increased cardiovascular risk [53]. For example, very low-calorie diets, liquid protein diets, and starvation have all been associated with prolongation of the QTc interval. In addition, liquid protein diets have been associated with potentially life-threatening arrhythmias documented on 24 hour Holter monitoring [54]. In addition, some medications have resulted in cardiac valve disorders and have been removed from the market including fenfluramine and dexfenfluramine. In addition, sibutramine has been associated with high blood pressure and should not be utilized in individuals with pre-existing hypertension.

12.8 DOES TREATMENT OF OBESITY DECREASE THE RISK OF CORONARY HEART DISEASE?

There is less currently available information on long-term effects of weight loss on CHD itself rather than on its risk factors. The Look AHEAD Trial, for example, did demonstrate that individuals who lost 5%–7% of their weight did achieve reduction in risk factors for CHD, but not in CHD itself [55]. The Cancer Prevention Study, which is a long-term study of over 750,000 women, demonstrated that obesity-related health conditions such as T2DM and hypertension in individuals who achieve potential weight loss experience a 9% reduction in CHD mortality.

It should also be noted that controversy exists about cardiovascular risk related to numerous cycles of weight loss and weight gain (weight cycling). Framingham data suggested that individuals who weight cycle may increase their risk of heart disease [56]. However, a meta-analysis conducted by the National Task Force on Prevention and Treatment of Obesity achieved the opposite conclusion that weight cycling did not increase the risk of CHD [57].

- *Role of abdominal obesity*: A number of studies have demonstrated that central (abdominal) obesity confers additional risks of CHD in addition to elevated BMI. This appears to be due to the fact that adipose tissue in the abdominal region is more metabolically active than the hips, thighs, or buttocks [58,59]. Waist circumference has largely replaced waist-to-hip ratio as a means of estimating abdominal fat. Abdominal fat is considered a core component of MetS which is comprised of a cluster in risk factors for CHD and represents a potent risk for CHD [60–62].

12.9   THE ROLE OF WEIGHT GAIN AS A RISK FACTOR FOR CHD

It should be noted that adult weight gain is also associated with CHD independent of obesity [63]. In the Nurses' Health Trial, weight gain between the age of 18 to midlife was associated in a linear fashion with increased risk of CHD. Women who gained between 5 and 7.9 kg during this stage of life increased their risk of CHD by 1.25 times. Those who gained ≥20 kg increased their risk of CHD by 2.65 times [64]. Significant weight gain after age 21 has also been correlated with increased risk of CHD in men in the U.S. Male Professional Follow-up Study [64]. Weight gain during adult years is also associated with increased risk of hypertension and stroke as well as T2DM.

- *Childhood obesity*: This chapter does not focus on childhood obesity per se (See Chapter 10). However, it should be noted that the earliest changes of atherosclerosis may be apparent as early as age five in children with obesity. Moreover, the prevalence of childhood obesity has dramatically increased in the United States as well as risk factors for CHD, T2DM, and MetS.

12.10   CLINICAL ASSESSMENT OF INDIVIDUALS WITH OBESITY

- *History and physical examination*: As discussed in Chapter 4, a history of weight should be taken in any individual with obesity to determine at what stage in life weight gain occurred. A physical examination may be difficult in an individual with obesity and manifestations of cardiovascular pathophysiology may be underestimated. However, there are certain tests that are particularly valuable in individuals with obesity from a CHD risk factor standpoint.
- *Electrocardiogram*: The electrocardiogram (ECG) in individuals with obesity may be difficult to interpret because of increased distance between the electrodes and the heart due to excessive pannus [65,66]. A variety of changes in ECG may occur with increasing obesity. These include low voltage, left access deviation, and non-specific SD and T wave flattening, particularly in the inferior and lateral leads. Dramatic elevation of ST segments may occur due to horizontal displacement of the heart. Voltage criteria for either left atrial abnormality or LVH are common findings. False positive criteria for inferior myocardial infarction may also be present which is also thought to be due to diagrammatic elevations [67].
- *Echocardiography*: Echocardiography may be useful in individuals with obesity to help ascertain cardiac status [68]. Both chamber size and wall thickness as well as a variety of left ventricular indices may be derived from echocardiography.
- *Assessment of CHD with imaging techniques*: Various imaging techniques to assess CHD may also be valuable in patients with obesity, particularly those with risk factors for CHD. Due to impaired exercise tolerance,

dipyridamole thallium scans [69] may be utilized to evaluate the presence of ischemic heart disease. Esophageal echocardiography may be useful as well. If heart cauterization is contemplated in individuals, the use of percutaneous radial approach may be most appropriate to minimize the risk of bleeding complications from a femoral approach [70].

12.11 TREATMENT OF OBESITY IN CLINICAL PRACTICE

Physician recommendation for behavioral change has been documented in a number of instances to be a powerful motivator and result in significant clinical improvements. However, in the area of obesity as a risk factor for cardiovascular disease, medical involvement appears to have been less than optimal. In a national survey of 2,000 adults with a BMI ≥25, only 22% of males and 39% of females ever received counseling about their weight [71].

There are many reasons why physician involvement in this important area of risk factor reduction for CHD in individuals with obesity may be lacking. Perhaps physicians underestimate the interaction between obesity and other risk factors for heart disease. Lack of reimbursement from insurance for counseling related to obesity has often been cited as a reason for physician lack of counseling in this area.

It has also been argued that physician reluctance to treat obesity may be due to a lack of demonstrated efficacy for the long-term treatment. Unfortunately, physicians may also share negative stereotyping of obesity as a lack of discipline or willpower. It is hoped that as scientific understandings for obesity as a chronic disease and a risk factor for CHD develop more physicians will become involved in treating obesity to lower the risk of CHD.

- *Vital signs of obesity*: One way to start treating obesity is to take the vital signs of obesity. Most physicians currently take the weight of their patients. However, BMI and waist circumference are also important variables. Once BMI is measured, physicians can then counsel patients on how BMI relates to the risk of various chronic diseases including CHD. More detail on this is found in Chapter 4.
- *Lifestyle management of obesity*: There is no longer any serious question that lifestyle changes play an important role in the prevention and management of various diseases. Lifestyle modalities include improved nutrition, increased physical activity, and behavioral modification [72]. Caloric restriction is a mainstay for the nutritional approach to weight loss. (See Chapter 6 for more detail.) Increased physical activity has also been demonstrated to confer multiple benefits for both short- and long-term weight loss. Physical activity is particularly important for the maintenance of weight loss and may, in addition, play an important role in the loss of abdominal fat and also long-term adherence to weight loss strategies. (See also Chapter 5 for more detail.)

  Behavioral strategies for weight loss has clearly been demonstrated to play a positive role in the overall approach to weight loss and maintenance of weight loss. Of course, both improved nutrition and physical activity are behaviors. However, there is much more information available on behavioral change for weight loss and maintenance of weight loss. This is discussed in more detail in Chapter 7.

Issues of maintenance of weight loss are often misunderstood in the medical community. The National Weight Control Registry, which has over 5,000 individuals who have lost a significant amount of weight and kept it off for at least a year, has shown that individuals who adopt daily strategies of monitoring their nutrition and participating in regular physical activity are highly successful both in short- and long-term weight loss. Moreover, the Look AHEAD Trial and the DPP Trial have shown that individuals can maintain a weight loss of 5%–7% of body weight in follow up for over 4 years.

- *Pharmacologic therapy for obesity*: A number of pharmacological modalities are available for the treatment of obesity. These are discussed in detail in Chapter 8. Pharmaceutical agents need to be used in conjunction with lifestyle measures and appear to have synergistic effects when used with these practices.
- *Coronary artery disease revascularization procedures in individuals with obesity*: Obese individuals tend to have a high percentage of multi-vessel coronary artery disease, but no more severity of disease than normal individuals in one study of heart catheterization. However, it should be noted that patients with obesity have been shown to have a higher instance of multiple postoperative complications following coronary artery bypass grafting (CABG) than lower weight individuals [73]. Individuals with obesity are particularly at risk for a thromboembolic disease and should receive an aggressive approach to deep venous thrombosis prophylactics.
- *Bariatric surgery*: Bariatric surgery has been demonstrated to be highly efficacious for reducing risk factors for CVD and T2DM in individuals with morbid obesity. Indications for bariatric surgery vary from institution to institution. These issues and other issues related to bariatric surgery are discussed in detail in Chapter 9.

12.12 SUMMARY/CONCLUSIONS

There are multiple, strong, and independent links between obesity and CHD. Obesity is also associated with multiple risk factors for CHD including hypertension, dyslipidemias, T2DM, and MetS.

The clustering of risk factors that occurs in conditions such as MetS is common in people who develop obstructive atherosclerosis. Weight loss provides an attractive option for simultaneously treating multiple risk factors for CHD. Physicians should be aware of the multiple links between obesity and heart disease and emphasize not only the treatment of obesity itself, but also how this treatment reduces associated cardiac risk factors.

CLINICAL APPLICATIONS

- Obesity is an independent risk factor for coronary heart disease.
- Obesity is also associated with multiple other risk factors for CHD including hypertension, dyslipidemias, T2DM, and MetS.

- Clinicians should emphasize to patients with obesity and overweight these linkages.
- Abdominal obesity is also particularly linked to an increased risk of heart disease.
- Clinicians should take the vital signs of obesity which include not only weight but also body mass index and waist circumference when they counsel patients about the link between obesity and heart disease.

REFERENCES

1. Rippe J. Lifestyle medicine: The health promoting power of daily habits and practices. *Am J Lifestyle Med.* 2018;13:6.
2. Stone N., Robinson J., Lichtenstein A., et al. 2013 ACC/AHA guideline on the treatment of blood cholesterol to reduce atherosclerotic cardiovascular risk in adults: A report of the American College of Cardiology/American Heart Association Task Force on Practice Guidelines. *Circulation.* 2014;129 (25 suppl 2):S1–S45.
3. Lloyd-Jones D., Hong Y., Labarthe D., et al. American Heart Association Strategic Planning Task Force and Statistics Committee. Defining and setting national goals for cardiovascular health promotion and disease reduction: The American Heart Association's strategic impact goal through 2020 and beyond. *Circulation.* 2010;121:586–613.
4. US Department of Health and Human Services; US Department of Agriculture. Dietary guidelines for Americans, 2015–2020. 8th ed. http://health.Gov/dietaryguidelines/2015/guidelines/. Published December 2015. Accessed August 26, 2020.
5. Mozaffarian D., Appel L., Van Horn L. Components of a cardioprotective diet: New insights. *Circulation.* 2011;123:2870–2891.
6. Estruch R., Ros E., Salas-Salvadó J., et al. PREDIMED study investigators. Primary prevention of cardiovascular disease with a Mediterranean diet. *N Engl J Med.* 2013;368:1279–1290.
7. Chiuve S.E., McCullough M.L., Sacks F.M., Rimm E.B. Healthy lifestyle factors in the primary prevention of coronary heart disease among men: Benefits among users and nonusers of lipid-lowering and antihypertensive medications. *Circulation.* 2006;114:160–167.
8. American Heart Association. Council on Lifestyle and Cardiometabolic Health. https://professional.heart.org/professional/MembershipCouncils/ScientificCouncils/UCM_322856_Council-on-Lifestyle-and-Cardiometabolic-Health.jsp. Accessed September 19, 2018.
9. Eckel R., Jakicic J., Ard J., et al. 2013 AHA/ACC guideline on lifestyle management to reduce cardiovascular risk: A report of the American College of Cardiology/American Heart Association task force on practice guidelines. *Circulation.* 2014;129(25 suppl 2):S76–S99.
10. American Heart Association Nutrition Committee, Lichtenstein A.H., Appel L.J., et al. Diet and lifestyle recommendations revision 2006: A scientific statement from the American Heart Association Nutrition Committee. *Circulation.* 2006;114:82–96.
11. Despres J.P. Abdominal obesity as important component of insulin-resistance syndrome. *Nutrition.* 1993;9:452–459.
12. National Center for Health Statistics. United States, 2016: With Chartbook on Long-Term Trends in Health. Hyattsville, MD: National Center for Health Statistics; 2017.
13. Jensen M., Ryan D., Apovian C. 2013 AHA/ACC/TOS guideline for the management of overweight and obesity in adults: A report of the American College of Cardiology/American Heart Association Task Force on practice guidelines and the obesity society. *J Am Coll Cardiol.* 2014;63(25 pt B):2985–3023.

14. Look AHEAD Research Group, Wing R., Bolin, P. Cardiovascular effects of intensive lifestyle intervention in type 2 diabetes. *N Engl J Med.* 2013;369:145–154.
15. Lesser G., Deutsch S. Measurement of adipose tissue blood flow and perfusion in man by uptake of 85Kr. *J Appl Physiol.* 1967;23:621–630.
16. Oberg B., Rosell S. Sympathetic control of consecutive vascular sections in canine subcutaneous adipose tissue. *Acta Physiol Scand.* 1967;71:47–56.
17. Wajchenberg B. Subcutaneous and visceral adipose tissue: Their relation to the metabolic syndrome. *Endocr Rev* 2000;21:697–738.
18. Hotamisligil G., Arner P., Caro J. et al. Increased adipose tissue expression of tumor necrosis factor-alpha in human obesity and insulin resistance. *J Clin Invest* 1995;95:2409–2415.
19. Lundgren C., Brown S., Nordt T., et al. Elaboration of type-1 plasminogen activator inhibitor from adipocytes: A potential pathogenetic link between obesity and cardiovascular disease. *Circulation.* 1996;93:106–110.
20. Yudkin J., Stehouwer C., Emeis J., et al. C-reactive protein in healthy subjects: Associations with obesity, insulin resistance, and endothelial dysfunction: a potential role for cytokines originating from adipose tissue? *Arterioscler Thromb Vasc Biol.* 1999;19:972–978.
21. Karpe F., Fieding V., Ilie V. et al. Monitoring adipose tissue blood flow in man: A comparison between the xenon washout method and microdialysis. *Int J Obes.* 2002;26:1–5.
22. Cigolini M., Targher G., Bergamo A., et al. Visceral fat accumulation and its relation to plasma hemostatic factors in healthy men. *Arterioscler Thromb Vasc Biol.* 1996;16:368–374.
23. Mohamed-Ali V., Goodrick S., Rawesh A., et al. Subcutaneous adipose tissue releases interleukin-6, but not tumor necrosis factor-alpha, in vivo. *J Clin Endocrinol Metab.* 1997;82:4196–4200.
24. Alpert M. Obesity cardiomyopathy: Pathophysiology and evolution of the clinical syndrome. *Am J Med Sci.* 2001;321:225–236.
25. Kaltman A., Goldring R. Role of circulatory congestion in the cardiorespiratory failure of obesity. *Am J Med.* 1976;60:645–653.
26. Sasson Z., Rasooly Y., Gupta R., et al. Left atrial enlargement in healthy obese: Prevalence and relation to left ventricular mass and diastolic function. *Can J Cardiol.* 1996;12:257–263.
27. Alpert M., Lambert C., Panayiotou H., et al. Relation of duration of morbid obesity to left ventricular mass, systolic function, and diastolic filling, and effect of weight loss. *Am J Cardiol.* 1995;76:1194–1197.
28. Hubert H., Feinleib M., McNamara P., et al. Obesity as an independent risk factor for cardiovascular disease: A 26-year follow-up of participants in the Framingham heart study. *Circulation.* 1983;67:968–977.
29. Bassuk S., Manson J. Lifestyle and risk of cardiovascular disease and type 2 diabetes in women: A review of the epidemiologic evidence. *Am J Lifestyle Med.* 2008;3:191–213.
30. McGill H., Jr. Fatty streaks in the coronary arteries and aorta. *Lab Invest.* 1968;18:560–564.
31. Skalen K., Gustafsson M., Rydberg E., et al. Subendothelial retention of atherogenic lipoproteins in early atherosclerosis. *Nature.* 2002;417:750–754.
32. Stamler J. Epidemiologic findings on body mass and blood pressure in adults. *Ann Epidemiol.* 1999;4:347–362.
33. Fagerberg B., Berglund A., Anderson O., et al. Weight reduction versus antihypertensive drug therapy in obese men with high blood pressure: Effects upon plasma insulin levels and association with changes in blood pressure and serum lipids. *J Hypertens.* 1992;10:1053–1061.

34. Stepniakowski K., Egan B. Additive effects of obesity and hypertension to limit venous volume. *Am J Physiol.* 1995;268:R562–R568.
35. Mokdad A., Ford E., Bowman B., et al. Prevalence of obesity, diabetes, and obesity-related health risk factors, 2001. *JAMA* 2003;289(1):76–79.
36. Field A., Coakley E., Must A., et al. Impact of overweight on the risk of developing common chronic diseases during a 10-year period. *Arch Intern Med.* 2001;161(13):1581–1586.
37. Denke M., Sempos C. Grundy S. Excess body weight: An unrecognized contribution to high blood pressure cholesterol levels in While American women. *Arch Intern Med.* 1993;153:1093–1103.
38. Denke M., Sempos C., Grundy S. Excess body weight: An unrecognized contribution to high blood pressure cholesterol levels in While American women. *Arch Intern Med.* 1994;154:401–410.
39. Nakajima T., Fujioka S., Tokunaga K., et al. Correlation of intraabdominal fat accumulation and left ventricular performance in obesity. *Am J Cardiol.* 1989;64:369–373.
40. Hansson P., Eriksson H., Welin L., et al. Smoking and abdominal obesity: risk factors for venous thromboembolism among middle-aged men: The study of men born in 1913. *Arch Intern Med.* 1999;159:1886–1890.
41. Kannel W., Plehn J., Cupples L. Cardiac failure and sudden death in the Framingham study. *Am Heart J.* 1988;115:869–875.
42. Peterson H., Rothschild M., Weinberg C., et al. Body fat and the activity of the autonomic nervous system. *N Engl J Med.* 1988;318:1077–1083.
43. Strollo P., Rogers R. Obstructive sleep apnea. *N Engl J Med.* 1996;334:99–104.
44. Stamler R., Stamler J., Gosch F., et al. Primary Prevention of hypertension by nutritional-hygienic means: Final report of a randomized, controlled trial. *JAMA.* 1989;262:1801–1807.
45. Hypertension Prevention Trial Research Group. The hypertension prevention trial: Three year effects of dietary changes on blood pressure. *Arch Inter Med.* 1990;150:153–162.
46. Trials of Hypertension Prevention Collaborative Research Group. The effects of non-pharmacologic interventions on blood pressure of persons with high normal levels: Results of the Trials of Hypertension Prevention, Phase I. *JAMA.* 1992;267:1213–1220.
47. National High Blood Pressure Education Program Working Group. National high blood pressure education program working group report on primary prevention of hypertension. *Arch Intern Med.* 1993;153:186–208.
48. Katzel L., Bleeker E., Colman E., et al. Effects of weight loss vs aerobic exercise training on risk factors for coronary heart disease to healthy, obese, middle-aged and older men. *JAMA* 1995;274:1915–1921.
49. Knowler W., Barrett-Connor E., Fowler S.E., et al. Reduction in the incidence of type 2 diabetes with lifestyle intervention or metformin. *N Engl J Med.* 2002;346(6):393–403.
50. Tuomilehto J., Lindstrom J., Eriksson J.G., et al. Prevention of type 2 diabetes mellitus by changes in lifestyle among subjects with impaired glucose tolerance. *N Engl J Med.* 2001;344(18):1343–1350.
51. Dattilo A., Kris-Etherton P. Effects of weight reduction on blood lipids and lipoproteins: A meta-analysis. *Am J Clin Nutr.* 1992;56:320–328.
52. Himeno E., Nishino K., Nakashima Y., et al. Weight reduction regresses left ventricular mass regardless of blood pressure level in obese subjects. *Am Heart J.* 1996;131:313–319.
53. Isner J., Sours H., Paris A., et al. Sudden, unexpected death in avid dieters using the liquid-protein-modified fast diet. Observations in 17 patients and the role of the prolonged QT interval. *Circulation.* 1979;60:1401–1412.
54. Pringle T., Scobie I., Murray R., et al. Prolongation of the QT interval during therapeutic starvation: A substrate for malignant arrhythmias. *Int J Obes.* 1983;7:253–261.

55. Ryan D., Espeland M., Foster G., et al. Look AHEAD (Action for Health in Diabetes): Design and methods for a clinical trial of weight loss for the prevention of cardiovascular disease in type 2 diabetes. *Control Clin Trials* 2003;24(5):610–628.
56. Hamm P., Shekelle R., Stamler J. Large fluctuations in body weight during young adulthood and 25 year risk of coronary death in men. *Am J Epidemiol* 1989;129:312–318.
57. National Task Force on the Prevention and Treatment of Obesity. Weight cycling. *JAMA.* 1994;272:1196–1202.
58. Despre J. Dyslipidemia and obesity. *Balliere Clin Endocrinol Met* 1994;8:629–660.
59. Despres J. Abdominal obesity as important component of insulin-resistance syndrome. *Nutrition.* 1993;4:452–459.
60. Ford E., Giles W., Dietz W. Prevalence of the metabolic syndrome among US adults: Findings from the third National Health and nutrition examination survey. *JAMA.* 2002;287(3):356–359.
61. Poirier P., Despres J. Waist circumference, visceral obesity, and cardiovascular risk. *J Cardiopulm Rehabil.* 2003;23:161–169.
62. Hansen B. The metabolic syndrome X. *Ann N Y Acad Sci.* 1999;892:1–24.
63. Willett W., Manson J., Stampfer M., et al. Weight, weight change, and coronary heart disease in women. Risk within the 'normal' weight range. *JAMA.* 1995;273(6):461–465.
64. Rexrode K., Hennekens C., Willett W., et al. A Prospective study of body mass index, weight change, and risk of stroke in women. *JAMA.* 1997;227:1539–1545.
65. Eisenstein I., Edelstein J., Sarma R., et al. The electrocardiogram in obesity. *J Electrocardiol.* 1982;15:115–118.
66. Master A., Oppenheimer E. A study of obesity: Circulatory, roentgen-ray and electrocardiographic investigations. *JAMA.* 1929;92:1652–1656.
67. Alpert M., Terry B., Cohen M., et al. The electrocardiogram in morbid obesity. *Am J Cardiol.* 2000;85:908–910.
68. Alpert M., Kelly D. Value and limitations of echocardiography assessment of obese patients. *Echocardiography.* 1986;3:261–272.
69. Ferraro S., Perrone-Filardi P., Desiderio A., et al. Left ventricular systolic and diastolic function in severe obesity: A radionuclide study. *Cardiology.* 1996;87:347–353.
70. McNulty P., Ettinger S., Field J., et al. Cardiac catheterization in morbidly obese patients. *Catheter Cardiovasc Interv.* 2002;56:174–177.
71. X-Factor Study, New York: Louis Harris and Associates, Inc., 1997.
72. Lem M., Wing R., McGuire M. et al. A descriptive study of individuals successful at long-term maintenance of substantial weight loss. *Am J Clin Nutr.* 1997;66:239–346.
73. Gruberg L., Weissman J., Waksman R. et al. The impact of obesity on the short-term and long-term outcomes after percutaneous coronary intervention: The obesity paradox? *J Am Coll Cardiol* 2002;39:578–584.

13 Obesity and Diabetes

James M. Rippe, MD
Rippe Lifestyle Institute
University of Massachusetts Medical School

CONTENTS

DOI: 10.1201/9781003099116-15

13.1   INTRODUCTION

Obesity has been clearly linked to an increased risk of developing type 2 diabetes (T2DM) as well as cardiovascular disease (CVD) through dysregulation of a variety of endocrine and inflammatory mechanisms, although the specific role of the mechanisms in the pathogenesis of T2DM remains incompletely understood and this is an area of considerable research. The mechanisms that link obesity, insulin resistance, and T2DM are central to the development of strategies toward the prevention and treatment of insulin resistance.

13.2   PREVALENCE OF OBESITY PANDEMIC

13.2.1   OBESITY-ASSOCIATED MORBIDITY AND MORTALITY

As described in multiple chapters throughout this book, overweight and obesity are defined as excessive or abnormal fat accumulation which may impair health. There are many mechanisms for estimating or measuring excessive adiposity (see also Chapters 3 and 4). In large epidemiologic studies, the typical measurement utilized to measure overweight and obesity is body mass index (BMI) which is weight in kilograms divided by height in meters (kg/m^2). BMI, utilizing World Health Organization (WHO), criteria defines "overweight" as a BMI greater than or equal 25 kg/m^2 and less than 30 kg/m^2 and obesity is a BMI equal to more than 30 kg/m^2 [1]. The prevalence of both overweight and obesity has increased dramatically in the last 40 years around the world. It is now estimated that there are over 2.1 billion individuals with obesity worldwide.

13.3   INSULIN RESISTANCE AND DIABETES: PATHOPHYSIOLOGY, SYMPTOMS, ASSESSMENT, AND ASSOCIATED COMPLICATIONS

13.3.1   OBESITY AND INSULIN RESISTANCE

Obesity-associated insulin resistance is a major risk factor for T2DM and CVD. Multiple endocrine and inflammatory markers have been demonstrated to be dysregulated in obesity (see also Chapter 2).

The influence of obesity on the risk of T2DM is determined not only by the degree of obesity (increased total fat mass) but by where fat accumulates. Increased upper body fat including visceral adiposity as reflected in increased abdominal girth is associated with metabolic syndrome (MetS), T2DM, and CVD [2,3].

Fat tissue dysfunction in obesity is characterized by an altered capacity to store lipids and enhanced adipose tissue inflammation both of which play crucial roles in the development of insulin resistance and T2DM [4].

In contrast, subcutaneous (SC) fat appears to lack the physiologic effects of visceral fat and functions simply as more of a neutral storage location.

In addition to body fat distribution, some evidence suggests that subtypes of adipose tissue are functionally distinct and may also affect glucose homeostasis. Adult humans have a limited amount of brown fat cells which play a role in thermogenesis and potentially influence energy expenditure and obesity susceptibility [5]. Brown adipose tissue (BAT), in contrast to white adipose tissue (WAT), is involved in energy dissipation rather than storage. In addition, adipose tissue is composed of heterogeneous cell types. For example, immune cells within adipose tissue contribute to systemic metabolic processes.

It appears that the main mechanisms that link obesity to insulin resistance and pre-disposal to T2DM include increased production of adipokines/cytokines including TNPK resistin and retinol-binding protein 4 (RBP4) that contribute to insulin resistance as well as reduced levels of adiponectin. In addition, ectopic fat deposition, particularly in liver but also in skeletal muscle which leads to dysmetabolic sequelae mitochondrial dysfunction, contributes to insulin resistance [6–10]. Some research suggests that mitochondrial dysfunction could be one of the most important underlying defects linking obesity to T2DM through the mechanism of decreasing insulin sensitivity and compromising beta-cell function.

13.3.2 MECHANISMS OF PROGRESSIVE B-CELL DYSFUNCTION IN OBESE INDIVIDUALS

Both T2DM and impaired glucose tolerance (IGT) have shown a reduction of both insulin secretion and insulin sensitivity [11–13]. One of the main mechanisms that cause this is the increased supply of fatty acids into circulation. Persistent positive energy balance is associated with increased storage of triglycerides which expands adipose depots and increases the proportion of hypertrophied adipocytes. Large adipocytes are less sensitive to the antilipolytic action of insulin, causing an increase in the liberation and turnover of fatty acids.

These fatty acids can then be taken up by liver and muscle where they are used in competition with glucose as a source of energy. Thus, the imbalance between glucose and fatty acid availability causes an increased availability of fatty acids and their oxidation reduces the utilization of glucose. Fatty acid metabolites also impair the post-receptor pathway of intracellular insulin signaling and decrease insulin-stimulated glucose transport in the muscle. Hyperinsulinemia is the first response of the beta cell to obesity. In turn, a reduced insulin action causes an upregulation on insulin secretion in order to maintain normoglycemia [14]. Obese normoglycemic individuals have both increased beta-cell mass and function. Factors predisposing to beta-cell decompensation could be either primarily genetic or epigenetic. The exact mechanism that causes this decompensation remains under research and is debated. At the current time, the known genes are estimated to predict T2DM by 15%. This low predictive power may reflect the high importance of environmental factors.

13.4 MECHANISMS LINKING OBESITY AND INSULIN RESISTANCE

13.4.1 ADIPOSE TISSUE MACROPHAGES: A LINK BETWEEN OBESITY-ASSOCIATED INFLAMMATION AND INSULIN RESISTANCE

Overall adipocyte function represents an important regulator of systemic insulin sensitivity [15]. Adipocytes produce substantial amounts of pro-inflammatory cytokines and chemokines including IL-6, and TNF-α [16]. In animal studies, the main contributor to inflammatory molecules is largely macrophages in adipose tissue. Due to its considerable size, adipose tissue and the macrophages present there are important regulators of systemic inflammation and insulin sensitivity in the obese [17].

Macrophages typically respond to signals concerning cellular damage or death. Hypertrophied adipocytes increase the likelihood of cell death which elicits an inflammatory response including infiltration of macrophages [18]. This type of macrophage infiltration is seen in obese individuals but not in lean counterparts. Macrophages in adipose tissue increase circulating concentrations of pro-inflammatory cytokines such as c-reactive protein (CRP) and adipokines which may contribute to insulin resistance. It has been suggested that cytokines promote insulin resistance by attracting macrophages into adipocytes, and once inside the adipose tissue, the macrophages secrete pro-inflammatory molecules that may lead to further recruitment of macrophages.

It should be emphasized that macrophages may not be the only or main source of inflammatory molecules and cytokines may not be the only cause of reducing insulin sensitivity in the obese state.

13.4.2   Toll-like Receptor: Linking Obesity and Inflammation

Toll-like Receptor 4 (TLR4) has been implicated as a potential link between obesity and diabetes. Obesity induces a marked elevation of free fatty acid (FFA) concentrations which may, in turn, trigger an inflammatory response in macrophages and adipocytes [15]. Saturated FFA may activate macrophage-like cells through the TLR4 pathway. Thus TLR4 may act as a sensor of increased FFA levels that ultimately leads to an inflammatory response and insulin-desensitizing actions. High-fat diets also may create a state of endotoxemia which causes hepatic insulin resistance resulting in fasting hyperglycemia and insulinemia as well as weight gain and adipose tissue inflammation.

13.4.3   Molecular Dysregulation Associated with Lipid Oversupply

T2DM is associated with obesity-induced insulin resistance. Insulin resistance represents a state where peripheral tissues fail to increase whole-body glucose disposal in response to insulin action. The two tissues most responsible for glucose clearance from the blood, liver, and muscle demonstrate reduced insulin-stimulated glucose uptake and metabolism contributing to the elevation of insulin resistance. This occurs particularly when the lipid supply is increased which is what happens in obesity.

According to the theory of Randle, accumulated fatty acids may hamper insulin-stimulated glucose uptake, particularly in muscle. In obesity-related lipid oversupply, intracellular glucose uptake is impaired as its utilization by inactivating some key glycolytic enzymes [19]. Insulin resistance in peripheral tissues and particularly skeletal muscle may be caused by or impaired by GLUT4 translocation or impaired insulin signaling.

What causes the intracellular fat accumulation in peripheral tissue such as skeletal muscle?

This accumulation appears to be related to a depression of fatty acid oxidation and/or elevated FFA transport into the cells. The FFA oxidation is reduced and fatty acid concentration in skeletal muscle is substantially higher in moderately and severely obese individuals compared with healthy counterparts [20,21].

Obesity has been shown to increase the level of circulating lipids, a condition that may predispose to an increase in FFA clearance in peripheral tissues such as skeletal muscle in the insulin-resistant state. It is hypothesized that obesity-induced upregulation of intracellular or lipid intermediates due to increased fatty acid uptake, in turn, alters insulin signaling resulting in decreased glucose transport and insulin resistance.

13.4.4 Genetic Links between Obesity and Type 2 Diabetes

Research has demonstrated that monogenic obesity is a rare phenomenon. A number of genes and genetic variance may be related to both the pathophysiology of obesity and diabetes [22]. These genes may act by altering fat oxidation, fat storage, fat transport, glucose transport, and energy balance. All of these genes may play a significant role in human obesity and diabetes.

13.4.5 Endocrine Links between Obesity and Diabetes

Impaired Catecholamine-Induced Lipolysis in the Obese Insulin Resistant State: Cause or Consequence?

One of the main characteristics of obesity is fat accumulation in adipose tissue in the form of triglycerides resulting in excessive lipid outflow into the blood compartment. This increased fat overflow into the circulation may result in increased uptake by other non-adipose peripheral tissues such as liver, pancreas, and skeletal muscle. This is a phenomenon also known as ectopic fat storage. Adipose tissue lipolysis is mainly regulated by catecholamines and insulin [23]. In obesity, a number of research studies have reported a blunted catecholamine-induced lipolysis.

The regulation of skeletal muscle lipolysis differs from that of adipose tissue. The elevated intramuscular triglycerides (ITG) which occur in obesity have been associated with skeletal muscle resistance and reflect an impaired capacity to utilize fat as an energy substrate in the mitochondria. It is uncertain whether this blunted catecholamine lipolysis in obesity is a primary cause or a consequence of insulin resistance in the obese. In either case, the blunted lipolysis may be an important factor in the pathogenesis of obesity and T2DM.

13.4.6 Impaired Free Fatty Acid Utilization in Skeletal Muscle

In impaired skeletal muscle lipolysis, adults with obesity may exhibit a reduced potential for oxidation of free fatty acids in their skeletal muscles, which, in turn, leads to overall reduced skeletal muscle oxidative potential which, in turn, impairs resting metabolic rate [24,25]. This reduced capacity of skeletal muscle to handle fat in obesity and T2DM may be attributed to a variety of biochemical factors. In addition, mitochondrial transport of long-chained fatty acids has also been implicated in the etiology of reduced-fat oxygenation in skeletal muscle of obese and T2DM individuals. Since mitochondria are critically important in skeletal muscle fat oxidation potential, mitochondrial dysfunction may represent an integral part of the pathogenesis of insulin resistance in T2DM.

13.4.7 ADIPOKINES

Systemic mediators of adipocyte dysfunction include adipokines, FFAs, and inflammatory mediators. Adipokines, including adiponectin, leptin, resistin, and ghrelin, are circulating molecules produced by adipocytes that affect energy use and production. Adipokines appear central in the pathophysiology of obesity and its systemic health effects, including nonalcoholic fatty liver disease, insulin resistance, atherosclerosis, and T2DM [26–28]. In addition to their effects on energy use, adipokines influence the production of inflammatory mediators. For example, adiponectin inhibits the synthesis and actions of TNF-α. Leptin increases the synthesis of IL-6 and TNF-α by macrophages and also activates macrophages. Resistin increases TNF-α and IL-6 synthesis, and its expression is, in turn, increased by those cytokines.

The fact that obesity, which is a major risk factor for T2DM and T2DM itself are inflammatory conditions, has led researchers to explore whether inflammatory mediators predict the development of T2DM in populations at risk. Several studies have confirmed that the presence of inflammation predicts the development of T2DM. TNFα, for example, plays a key role in linking inflammation, insulin resistance, obesity, and T2DM through a variety of mechanisms. A consensus statement ranked the increased production of adipokines/cytokines including TNFα, resistance, and RBP4 that contribute to insulin resistance as well as reduced levels of adiponectin as among the three most distinct mechanisms that link obesity to insulin resistance and a predisposition to T2DM.

13.4.8 GLUCOCORTICOIDS

Augmented glucocorticoids may induce insulin resistance and T2DM by opposing the anti-gluconeogenic action of insulin in the hepatic tissue [29]. Although blood glucocorticoid concentration is almost physiological in the obese, adipose tissue may increase cortisol production by cortisone to cortisol through a variety of mechanisms. These increased glucocorticoid levels are observed in individuals with "apple-shaped" fat distribution compared to individuals with "pear-shaped" fat distribution. This had led to the suggestion that adipose tissue-derived cortisol reaches liver through the portal vein circulation and contributes to hepatic insulin resistance.

13.5 CELL-INTRINSIC MECHANISMS LINKING OBESITY TO DIABETES

13.5.1 ECTOPIC FAT STORAGE

When FFAs and other lipids are chronically elevated in the circulation (as happens in individuals with obesity), they may lead to ectopic fat storage as triglycerides are stored in liver and skeletal muscle [30]. Ectopic fat storage may contribute to the development of insulin resistance through a variety of mechanisms [31].

The clinical manifestations of obesity are not only associated with mechanisms by which fat is stored (i.e. adipocyte proliferation vs. adipocyte hypertrophy), but also where the fat is stored. The various fat depots have unique characteristics – these range from smaller fat depots that track with visceral fat (VAT) such as pericardial and buccal or larger fat depots like the superficial and deep abdominal superficial fat (SAT). Intra-abdominal fat includes omental and mesenteric (visceral) depots, both of which drain into the portal vein as well as perinephric fat, which drains into the systemic circulation.

Fat depots other than VAT have pathogenic potential. The reason that ectopic fat is present in obesity is that during positive caloric balance adipocytes are unable to store excess energy mostly in the form of triglycerides so circulating FFA are increased and accumulate in non-adipose tissue organs such as liver, muscle, pancreas, and blood vessels leading to abnormalities of glucose and lipid metabolism as well as high blood pressure.

The majority of circulating FFAs actually originated from the SAT because SAT is the largest fat depot constituting approximately 80% or more of total body fat [32,33]. Thus, while VAT is generally considered the most pathological fat depot, SAT fat storage is limited or impaired during positive caloric balance, and SAT dysfunction may adversely affect non-hepatic organs, resulting in lipotoxicity to muscle (causing insulin resistance) and pancreas (possibly reducing insulin secretion).

Thus, the characteristics of adipose tissue are more important than the amount of body fat in determining the risk of obesity-related metabolic disease. Insulin resistance is associated with increased fat-cell size and increased adipose tissue lipolytic activity, and the accumulation of ectopic fat in other organs, particularly liver, might be a marker of adipose tissue pathology.

13.5.2 OXIDATIVE STRESS

Oxidative stress represents an imbalance between the generation of reactive oxygen and nitrogen molecular reactive species (RONS) and the antioxidant defense reserves of the body or individual tissues) [34]. Oxidative stress has been associated with fat accumulation in both humans and animals. Most evidence indicates that oxidative stress is a consequence of insulin resistance-induced hyperglycemia and not a cause of T2DM.

13.5.3 MITOCHONDRIAL DYSFUNCTION

Advanced insulin resistance has been linked to a marked elevation in triacylglycerol concentration in both skeletal muscle and hepatic tissues probably due to ectopic fat accumulation [35]. Ectopic fat accumulation is associated with impairment in mitochondrial function which is manifested by reduced mitochondrial oxidative activity and ATP production. A number of research studies have suggested that impaired mitochondrial dysfunction may induce insulin resistance. This may, in turn, contribute to intracellular fat accumulation in muscle which impairs insulin signaling causing insulin resistance.

13.5.4 NEURAL MECHANISMS

There are reports suggesting that the brain accepts signals from the periphery regarding fatness level signaling to the brain regarding adipocytes mediated by hormones such as leptin and insulin whose levels in the circulation depend on body's fat mass [36–38]. Hyperglycemia and insulin resistance may result from a disruption of mechanisms regulating the circadian rhythms in the hypothalamus. These mechanisms may induce central adaptations which can lead to insulin sensitivity deregulation.

13.6 COMMON APPROACHES TO TREAT INSULIN RESISTANCE AND OBESITY

Diabetes is the twin pandemic related to the obesity pandemic. It is estimated that T2DM will reach 366 million cases worldwide by the year 2030 [39]. It is also important to understand that 20%–50% of diabetics have undiagnosed. T2DM also exerts an enormous expenditure on the health care system as well as the medical issues for individuals.

Lifestyle interventions including physical activity, nutritional strategies, and other behavioral approaches have been studied and advanced as therapeutic modalities for humans at high risk for developing T2DM. The goal of these strategies is to lower the incidence of obesity and T2DM, as well as to reduce cardiovascular morbidity and mortality.

13.6.1 PHYSICAL ACTIVITY

One of the main reasons for the obesity pandemic is habitual physical inactivity as well as an abundance of energy-dense food particularly in industrialized countries that has resulted in the disturbance of the energy balance equation (See also Chapters 2 and 5).

If there is excess energy, human beings can easily convert this into adipose tissue TAG but humans have difficulty converting stored fat into energy if they are not physical active.

When obesity is combined with physical inactivity and overconsumption of high-calorie foods, there is clearly an elevated mortality risk, insulin resistance, and T2DM as described in the mechanisms already discussed in this chapter. Physical activity is perhaps the most important non-pharmacological treatment for the prevention and care of obesity, insulin resistance, and T2DM.

As outlined in the Physical Activity Guidelines for Americas 2018 Scientific Report, a minimum of 150 min/week of moderate intensity exercise is recommended for all adults [40]. Unfortunately, less than 25% of adults are achieving this level of regular physical activity (See also Chapter 5).

Physical activity carries multiple health benefits including enhancing glycemic control and endothelial function and reducing low-grade inflammation while improving cardiovascular conditioning and body composition. Physical activity in combination with energy restriction has been repeatedly shown to help achieve both weight loss and fat loss in adults with obesity. Exercise is particularly important for visceral fat loss. This is important since visceral adiposity is associated with an increased risk of insulin resistance.

As applied to the treatment of T2DM, regular physical activity may result in reduced hemoglobin A1c by as much as 0.8% [41,42]. Exercise also increases fat loss and reduces fasting blood lipids while improving high blood pressure and skeletal muscle oxidative capacity and mitochondrial function. VAT reductions may be responsible for the improvement in glycemic control in diabetics with exercise training.

With regard to the type of physical activity recommended, aerobic or cardiovascular exercise has typically been the main choice among exercise specialists for patients with obesity and T2DM patients. Resistance exercise has also been included in clinical guidelines for the prevention and treatment of T2DM but does not produce greater fat loss than aerobic exercise alone. However, the addition of resistance exercise training to aerobic may prevent or attenuate loss of skeletal muscle tissue during weight loss, thereby helping to maintain metabolic rate.

With regard to exercise training, most authoritative recommendations propose a range of 40%–80% of VO2 max in individuals with obesity, which corresponds to moderate intensity physical activity. Recently, high-intensity interval training (HIIT) has received considerable attention for its effects on individuals with obesity with metabolic syndrome symptoms (MetS) [43]. It has been reported that HIIT in individuals with obesity generates equal fat loss but greater improvement in insulin sensitivity and functional performance compared to moderate intensity continual physical activity in patients with MetS [44]. There is, however, no evidence regarding the effectiveness of HIIT on glycemic control. It should be noted that many individuals will find it difficult to maintain this kind of HIIT so it should be applied with caution to individuals with obesity who are insulin resistant.

With regard to the duration of physical activity, many clinical guidelines recommend at least 40 min of physical activity per training session and up to a total of 60 minutes. It appears that a greater duration of physical activity may be more beneficial for glycemic control and mitochondrial function. Recent information from the PAGA 2018 suggests that accumulated physical activity of much shorter duration per bout can also yield important health benefits.

13.6.2 NUTRITION

T2DM is a complex metabolic disease which is induced mainly through a combination of lifestyle factors (i.e. obesity, inactivity) in the context of a genetic predisposition. Nutrition therapy is an important part of diabetes prevention since it can reduce potential complications associated with hypertension and poor lipid or glycemic control [45]. Weight loss is recommended in the treatment of T2DM and insulin resistance since it improves glycemic control. In the later stages of T2DM, when insulin deficiency becomes more prominent than insulin resistance, weight loss may be less effective in respect to glycemic control. A number of plans have been put forth by the American Diabetes Association (ADA) for nutrition therapy both for obese and T2DM. For details concerning these recommendations, see Chapter 6.

13.6.3   IMPROVING INSULIN SENSITIVITY IN OBESITY WITH PHARMACOLOGICAL AGENTS

Pharmacologic agents should aim not only to weight loss but also particularly on the loss of fat mass, changes in the distribution of fat even without weight loss, and/or direct effects on adipose tissue dysfunction. Decreasing the amount of VAT can be accomplished through weight loss per se, loss of fat mass with an increase in fat-free mass (as seen with physical activity), or by inducing a shift in fat distribution from visceral to subcutaneous compartments. Diet-induced weight loss is an effective strategy for improving adipose tissue function but a minimum of 7% of weight loss is needed to improve many risk factors and at least 10% to improve plasma concentrations of adiponectin and lower inflammatory markers such as CRP [46].

13.6.4   AVAILABLE MEDICATIONS FOR WEIGHT LOSS

A variety of medicines are now available for weight loss. They include the following: (see Chapter 6 for more details) Orlistat (Orlistat is a lipase inhibitor that decreases intestinal fat absorption after meals).

Cannabinoid-1 (CB1) Receptor Antagonists. These receptors are widely dispersed throughout the body with high concentrations in areas of the brain. These receptors are also present in adipocytes. For this reason, a number of cannabinoid-1 receptor antagonists have been as weight loss medicines (See also Chapter 8 for a more complete list of available medications for weight loss and their affects).

13.6.5   OTHER NON-BEHAVIORAL TREATMENTS

13.6.5.1   Bariatric Surgery

Bariatric surgery is utilized as a strategy to reduce body weight and thereby ameliorate risk factors for cardiovascular disease. General guidelines for individuals who are potential candidates for bariatric surgery include those with a BMI greater than 30 km/m^2 and at least one risk factor for CVD or T2DM or BMI greater than 40 kg/m^2. On average, patients lose 14%–25% weight after bariatric surgery [47]. Bariatric surgery in some studies has also been shown to increase levels of adiponectin (See Chapter 9 for more details).

13.7   CONCLUSIONS

The global epidemic of obesity largely explains the dramatic rise in the incidence and prevalence of T2DM over the past 20 years. A number of research studies have identified links between obesity and T2DM involving inflammation, cytokines, insulin resistance, disrupted fatty acid metabolism, and cellular processes such as mitochondrial dysfunction. The interplay between obesity and diabetes is complex; however, effective weight loss in individuals with obesity will typically also improve risk factors for diabetes or make its control more possible.

CLINICAL APPLICATIONS

- Clinicians should be aware of the interplay between obesity and type 2 diabetes mellitus.
- The goal for obesity treatment should be not only weight loss but, in particular, visceral fat loss.
- Linkages between obesity and diabetes include inflammation, cytokines, insulin resistance, disruptive fatty acid metabolism, and mitochondrial dysfunction.
- All of these should be explored when treating obesity and/or type 2 diabetes mellitus.

REFERENCES

1. WHO criteria for Obesity by BMI - World Health Organization. Obesity: preventing and managing the global epidemic of obesity. Report of the WHO Consultation of Obesity. Geneva, 3–5 June 1997.
2. The Emerging Risk Factor Collaboration. Separate and combined associations of body-mass index and abdominal adiposity with cardiovascular disease: Collaborative analysis of 58 prospective studies. *Lancet.* 2011; 377:1085–95.
3. Montague C., O'Rahilly S. The perils of portliness: Causes and consequences of visceral adiposity. *Diabetes.* 2000; 49:883–93.
4. Goossens G. The role of adipose tissue dysfunction in the pathogenesis of obesity-related insulin resistance. *Physiol Behav.* 2008; 94:206–18.
5. Stephens M., Ludgate M., Rees A. Brown fat and obesity: The next big thing? *Clin Endocr.* 2011; 74(6):661–70.
6. Rube H., Lehrke M., Parhofer K., et al. Adipokines and insulin resistance. *Mol Med.* 2008; 14:741–51.
7. Antuna-Puente B., Feve B., Fellahi S., et al. Adipokines: The missing link between insulin resistance and obesity. *Diabetes Metab.* 2008; 34:2–11.
8. Graham T., Yang Q., Bluher M., et al. Retinol-binding protein 4 and insulin resistance in lean, obese, and diabetic subjects. *New Engl J Med.* 2006; 354:2552–63.
9. Sul H. Resistin/ADSF/FIZZ3 in obesity and diabetes. *Trends Endocrinol Metab.* 2005; 15:247–9.
10. Kadowaki T., Yamauchi T. Adiponectin and adiponectin receptors. *Endocr Rev.* 2005; 26:439–51.
11. Mitrakou A., Kelley D., Veneman T., et al. Contribution of abnormal muscle and liver glucose metabolism to postprandial hyperglycemia in non-insulin dependent diabetes mellitus. *Diabetes.* 1990; 39:1381–90.
12. Pimenta W., Mitrakou A., Jensen T., et al. Insulin secretion and insulin sensitivity in people with impaired glucose tolerance. *Diab Med.* 1996; 13(9 Suppl 6):S33–6.
13. Kahn S. The relative contributions of insulin resistance and beta-cell dysfunction to the pathophysiology of type 2 diabetes. *Diabetologia.* 2003; 46:3–19.
14. Turner R., Holman R., Matthews D., et al. Insulin deficiency and insulin resistance interaction in diabetes: Estimation of their relative contribution by feedback analysis from basal plasma insulin and glucose concentrations. *Metabolism.* 2019; 28:1086–96.
15. Zeyda M., Stulnig T. Obesity, inflammation, and insulin resistance: A mini-review. *Gerontology.* 2009; 55:379–86.
16. Hotamisligil G., Shargill N., Spiegelman B. Adipose expression of tumor necrosis factor-α: Direct role in obesity-linked insulin resistance. *Science.* 1993; 259:87–91.

17. Fain J. Release of interleukins and other inflammatory cytokines by human adipose tissue is enhanced in obesity and primarily due to the nonfat cells. *Vitam Horm.* 2006; 74:443–77.

18. Weisberg S., McCann D., Desai M., et al. Obesity is associated with macrophage accumulation in adipose tissue. *J Clin Invest.* 2003; 112:1796–808.

19. Randle P., Garland P., Hales C., et al. The glucose fatty-acid cycle. Its role in insulin sensitivity and the metabolic disturbances of diabetes mellitus. *Lancet.* 1963; 1:785–9.

20. Hulver M., Berggren J., Cortright R., et al. Skeletal muscle lipid metabolism with obesity. *Am J Physiol.* 2003; 284:E741–7.

21. MacLean P., Bower J., Vadlamudi S., et al. Lipoprotein subpopulation distributions in lean, obese, and type 2 diabetic women: A comparison of African and white Americans. *Obes Res.* 2000; 8:62–70.

22. Schmidt C., Gonzaludo N., Strunk S., et al. A meta-analysis of QTL for diabetes related traits in rodents. *Physiol Genomics,* 2008; 34:42–53.

23. Lafontan M., Langin L. Lipolysis and lipid mobilization in human adipose tissue. *Prog Lipid Res.* 2008; 48:275–97.

24. Pan D., Lillioja S., Kriketos A., et al. Skeletal muscle triglyceride levels are inversely related to insulin action. *Diabetes.* 1997; 46:983–8.

25. Zurlo F., Lillioja S., Esposito-Del Puente A., et al. Low ratio of fat to carbohydrate oxidation as predictor of weight gain: Study of 24-h RQ. *Am J Physiol.* 1990; 259:E650–E657.

26. Tilg H., Moschen A., Adipocytokines: Mediators linking adipose tissue, inflammation and immunity. *Nat Rev Immunol.* 2006; 6:772–83.

27. Arita Y., Kihara S., Ouchi N. Paradoxical decrease of an adipose-specific protein, adiponectin, in obesity. *Biochem Bioph Res Com.* 1999; 257:79–83.

28. Hotta K., Funahashi T., Arita Y., et al. Plasma concentrations of a novel, adipose-specific protein, adiponectin, in type 2 diabetic patients. *Arterioscl Thromb Vasc Biol.* 2000; 20:1595–9.

29. Seckl J. 11beta-hydroxysteroid dehydrogenases: Changing glucocorticoid action. *Curr Opin Pharmacol.* 2004; 4:597–602.

30. Qatanani M., Lazar M. Mechanisms of obesity-associated insulin resistance: Many choices on the menu. *Genes Dev.* 2007; 21:1443–55.

31. Unger R., Orci L. Lipotoxic diseases of nonadipose tissues in obesity. *Int J Obes Relat Metab Disord.* 2000; 24(Suppl. 4):S28–32.

32. Pasarica M., Xie H., Hymel D., et al. Lower total adipocyte number, but no evidence for small adipocyte depletion in patients with type 2 diabetes. *Diabetes Care.* 2009; 32:900–2.

33. Klein S. The case of visceral fat: Argument for the defense. *J Clin Invest.* 2004; 113:1530–2.

34. Halliwell B. Antioxidant characterization. Methodology and mechanism. *Biochem Pharmacol.* 1995; 49:1341–8.

35. Petersen K., Shulman G. Etiology of insulin resistance. *Am J Med.* 2006 119:S10–6.

36. Obici S., Feng Z., Arduini A., et al. Inhibition of hypothalamic carnitine palmitoyltransferase-1 decreases food intake and glucose production. *Nat Med.* 2003; 9:756–61.

37. Pocai A., Lam T., Obici S., et al. Restoration of hypothalamic lipid sensing normalizes energy and glucose homeostasis in overfed rats. *J Clin Invest.* 2006; 116:1081–91.

38. Seeley R., Woods S. Monitoring of stored and available fuel by the CNS: Implications for obesity. *Nat Rev Neurosci.* 2003; 4:901–9.

39. Wild S., Roglic G., Green A., et al. Global prevalence of diabetes: Estimates for the year 2000 and projections for 2030. *Diabetes Care.* 2004; 27(5):1047–53.

40. Physical Activity Guidelines for Americans 2018. 2nd edition. Accessed: August 26, 2020 https://health.gov/sites/default/files/2019-09/Physical_Activity_Guidelines_2nd_edition.pdf.

41. De Feyter H., Praet S., van den Broek N., et al. Exercise training improves glycemic control in long-standing insulin-treated type 2 diabetic patients. *Diabetes Care*. 2007; 30(10):2511–3.

42. Snowling N., Hopkins W. Effects of different modes of exercise training on glucose control and risk factors for complications in type 2 diabetic patients. *Diabetes Care*. 2006; 29(11):2518–27.

43. Schjerve I., Tyldum G., Tjonna A., et al. Both aerobic endurance and strength training programmes improve cardiovascular health in obese adults. *Clin Sci*. 2008; 115(9):283–93.

44. Tjonna A., Lee S., Rognmo O., et al. Aerobic interval training versus continuous moderate exercise as a treatment for the metabolic syndrome. *Circulation*. 2008; 118(4):346–54.

45. American Diabetes Association. Nutrition recommendations and interventions for diabetes. A Position Statement of the American Diabetes Association. *Diabetes Care*. 2008; 31(suppl 1):S61–S78.

46. Madsen E., Rissanen A., Bruun J., et al. Weight loss larger than 10% is needed for general improvement of levels of circulating adiponectin and markers of inflammation in obese subjects: A 3-year weight loss study. *Eur J Endocrinol*. 2008; 158:179–87.

47. Sjostrom L., Narbro K., Sjostrom, C., et al. Effects of bariatric surgery on mortality in Swedish obese subjects. *N Engl J Med*. 2007; 357:741–52.

14 Obesity and the Metabolic Syndrome

James M. Rippe, MD
Rippe Lifestyle Institute
University of Massachusetts Medical School

CONTENTS

14.1 INTRODUCTION

The metabolic syndrome (MetS), which is a grouping of physiologic variables, was actually identified in clinical practice almost a century ago by a Swedish physician who recognized that hypertension, hyperglycemia, and gout commonly occurred together [1]. The relationship between obesity, android adiposity, and the presence of hyperinsulinemia, hypertension, and elevated triglycerides has gained greater recognition in the past two decades with the advent of tests to reliably measure insulin and blood constituents.

The modern recognition of this syndrome in medicine and science can probably be dated to 1988 when Dr. Gerald Raeven introduced the term to describe the linkage between insulin resistance and hyperinsulinemia with underlying conditions to develop dyslipidemia, hypertension, and heightened cardiovascular disease (CVD) risk [2].

The rising prevalence of MetS has correlated with the surge in obesity rates [3–7]. This suggests that obesity contributes to the clustering of CVD risk factors. It is now widely recognized within the medical community that the clustering of

DOI: 10.1201/9781003099116-16

cardiovascular and metabolic risk factors is intricately connected to excess adiposity. This has laid the groundwork for the biological concept which is now known as MetS.

14.2 ELUSIVE DEFINITION OF METABOLIC SYNDROME

A wide variety of terms and definitions have been utilized to describe this clustering of risk factors. It is now generally agreed, however, that the clinical characteristics of MetS are increased waist circumference reflective of excess abdominal adiposity, impaired fasting glucose (IFG), elevated triglyceride concentrations, low high-density lipoprotein (HDL) cholesterol, and high blood pressure [8,9]. While many physicians still do not routinely diagnose MetS, it is clearly useful in terms of linking various metabolic conditions such as obesity, T2DM, and CVD risk. In fact, in the NCEP Guidelines (National Cholesterol Education Program), individuals with MetS are recommended to be treated as though they already have cardiovascular disease. Moreover, MetS is useful because it emphasizes in clinical practice the importance of primary prevention strategies.

In 2001, the National Cholesterol Education Program Adult Treatment Panel III (NCEP-ATP III) published a set of criteria for determining MetS [10]. The NCEP-ATP III approach required diagnosis for both insulin resistance and central obesity. These criteria which are the most widely used worldwide now concluded that if three of the five abnormalities were observed, MetS was present:

- Large waist circumference (>102 cm; >40 inches in men and >88 cm >35 inches in women)
- Impaired fasting glucose
- IFG (>100 mg/dl)
- Elevated triglycerides (>150 mg/dl)
- Elevated blood pressure (> 130 mg Hg/>85 mm/Hg)
- Low HDL cholesterol (<40 mg/dl for men and <50 mg/dl for women)

The clinical features of the metabolic syndrome as defined in the NCEP-ATP III guidelines are found in Table 14.1. Soon after the NCEP Guidelines were issued, the American Heart Association (AHA) and the National Heart Lung and Blood Institute (NHLBI) issued diagnostic criteria which were very similar to the NECP guidelines.

14.3 DESCRIBING THE METABOLIC SYNDROME
IN THE UNITED STATES

The prevalence of MetS varies considerably depending on the definition that is used [11–13]. The NCEP-ATP III criteria are the ones most frequently recognized in the United States to establish the prevalence of MetS and determine cardiometabolic risk.

Using these criteria, the prevalence of MetS increased from 23% to 27% in adult Americans aged 20 or older utilizing the NHANES data (1988–1994; 1999–2000). More recently Ford and Dietz [4,5] estimated higher rates of MetS (34.5%–39% of

TABLE 14.1

Clinical Features of the Metabolic Syndrome

Risk Factor	Defining Level
Abdominal obesity(waist circumference)	
Men	>102 cm (>40 in)
Women	>88 cm (>35 in)
HDL cholesterol	
Men	<40 mg/dl
Women	<50 mg/dl
Triglycerides	>150 mg/dl
Fasting glucose	>100 mg/dl
Blood pressure (systolic/diastolic)	>130 mmHg/>85 mmHg

HDL, high-density lipoprotein.

FROM: National Cholesterol Education Program (NCEP) ATPIII Criteria for the Metabolic Syndrome (MetS). US Department of Health and Human Services, NIH Document 01-3670. May 2001.

adults). This represents over 70 million adults living with MetS by NCEP-ATP III criteria.

Increases in overweight and obesity from the mid-1970s onward have correlated with the increased prevalence of MetS. Overweight and obesity greatly influence the prevalence of MetS since this condition occurs principally in individuals with obesity or overweight [14,15]. For example, using 1999–2004 NHANES data, 23.5% of normal weight individuals were found to have two or more cardiometabolic abnormalities when compared with 49.7% adults who are overweight and 69.3% of adults with obesity [16]. These are important findings given that according to Framingham data the majority of heart disease occurs in individuals who have two or more risk factors. In addition to age, ethnicity, and obesity, MetS is more prevalent in those who engage in little or no physical activity. MetS also occurs more frequently with greater carbohydrate consumption and reduced fiber intake.

14.4 CONTROVERSIES IN METS IN SCIENCE AND MEDICINE

The major controversy concerning MetS is whether insulin resistance and obesity are unifying causes of the syndrome [17,18]. It is estimated that only 48% of people with insulin resistance have MetS. This appears to be a result of the ability of physiologic processes to compensate for impaired insulin on glucose intake. On the other hand, 78% of patients who meet criteria for MetS diagnosis have insulin resistance [19,20]. This suggests that the underlying causes of MetS are more complex than simply insulin resistance or compensatory hyperinsulinemia.

With regard to obesity, there are between 29% and 35% of individuals with obesity who do not qualify for MetS and between 21% and 30% of normal weight individuals who would be defined as having MetS [21]. Therefore, although obesity does increase cardiometabolic risk, it does not consistently result in metabolic dysfunction.

Among those who feel that MetS is not useful in clinical practice, there is still a strong understanding that identifying the risk of CVD and T2DM is important. These clinicians feel that the diagnosis of MetS does not add anything to the diagnosis. On the other hand, proponents of MetS contend that clustering of risk factors that comprise MetS does not appear by random chance and that the clustering of these risk factors confers a significant risk of coronary heart disease (CHD), myocardial infarction, stroke, and T2DM. In addition, the issue arises of whether or not MetS offers greater predictive acuity than the sum of its individual components.

14.5 PREDICTING CARDIOMETABOLIC RISK FROM METS

There is widespread agreement that MetS predicts a higher risk of CVD and T2DM. In one meta-analysis of 87 studies involving 951,083 patients, overall CVD risk was 2.3 times greater than those with MetS [22]. In another meta-analysis of 37 longitudinal studies involving 172,573 patients, greater risk of CVD was reported with participants with MetS than those without the syndrome (RR = 1.78) [23].

In an analysis of 16 cohorts involved with 42,419 patients, MetS was consistently shown to have a strong association with incident T2DM [24]. Overall MetS is more strongly associated with incident T2DM than CVD outcomes. Those with MetS are at least twice as likely to develop CVD and even more likely to develop T2DM within the next decade [25–27]. To determine whether or not MetS is superior to predicting future CVD and T2DM than its components, findings remain inconclusive and are subject to an ongoing debate.

14.6 OBESITY AND THE ETIOLOGY OF INSULIN RESISTANCE AND METABOLIC SYNDROME

Insulin resistance in MetS and T2DM affects insulin signaling pathways differently. In skeletal muscle, insulin-mediated glucose uptake which counts for the disposal of up to 90% of insulin-mediated glucose is attenuated [28,29]. In adipose tissue, the insulin-mediated suppression of non-esterified fatty acid (NEFA) mobilization and secretion is dampened. This results in systemic metabolic dysfunction characterized by compensatory hyperinsulinemia, hyperglycemia, elevated NEFAs, and chronic low-grade inflammation.

Insulin resistance, relative hyperinsulinemia, and features of MetS are frequently exhibited in obese individuals with overt T2DM. CVD risk factors and clinically defined measures of atherosclerosis are more common and observed with greater intensity in obese versus normal weight individuals [30]. It should be noted that not all individuals with obesity develop insulin resistance or MetS. Thus, obesity is a poorly defined CVD risk factor which may present from otherwise apparently healthy individuals to exhibiting multiple risk factors, signs, or symptoms of cardiometabolic disease.

Some fat deposits such as gynoid or subcutaneous adipose tissue are thought to serve as a "metabolic sink" and may actually prevent the development of insulin resistance and MetS [31,32].

Visceral fat, however, is associated with insulin resistance and development of cardiovascular and metabolic dysfunction [33,34]. Visceral fat, in contrast to subcutaneous fat, increases the risk of hypertension and various components of CVD as well as mortality independent of total obesity. Excess fat may accumulate in sites that are not well suited to store fat such as the liver, skeletal and cardiac muscle, pancreas, and kidneys [35–37]. This additional fat burden within these tissues is "lipotoxic." That is because ectopic fat induces or greatly contributes to insulin resistance as well as disturbing glucose and lipid metabolism and contributing to inflammation and heightened oxidative stress.

Similar sequelae occur with visceral fat. In the liver, an oversupply of NEFA facilitates triglyceride synthesis and enhances the production of triglyceride-rich VLDL. Ectopic liver fat also potentiates the transfer of triglyceride from VDLD to HDL and results in the formation of small, dense LDL which more readily penetrates the vascular endothelium and is more susceptible to oxidative damage [38,39]. A reduction in HDL and altered HDL composition further impairs reverse cholesterol transport and contributes to dyslipidemia, vascular dysfunction, and atherosclerotic plaque burden. Thus, the molecular pathophysiology of obesity, insulin resistance, MetS, and related adverse cardiometabolic health outcomes is quite complex.

14.7 SCREENING AND EVALUATION FOR METS

Utilizing MetS in clinical screening may help classify patients that might otherwise be considered low risk using traditional risk factors such as age, sex, smoking, blood pressure, and cholesterol and may allow the clinician to consider the underlying cause of risk factor clustering [40]. This further allows the prescription of lifestyle behaviors that are known to have a powerful influence on cardiometabolic health (e.g. physical inactivity and poor diet).

As a practical matter, it is useful to identify and treat MetS in patients with obesity. This can be facilitated by utilizing one of the current MetS definitions such as that provided by NCEP-ATP III. This may then be followed up by calculating the near-term risk for CVD outcomes utilizing an established risk factor framework such as the Framingham Risk Score. Additions to the Framingham Risk Score [41] may include the use of BMI in younger individuals and measuring high sensitivity C reactive protein (hsCRP) as a marker of chronic inflammation as components of the overall risk with those who have intermediate or high risk 10 year Framingham scores. This approach will help the clinician formulate appropriate immediate treatment strategies as well as long-term management goals for patients with MetS.

14.8 TREATMENT AND MANAGEMENT OF METS

The goal of clinical management of MetS is to reduce the global risk of CVD, T2DM, and other metabolic diseases.

The current goals and recommendations for managing components of MetS are described in various consensus statements for dyslipidemia, high blood pressure, obesity, T2DM, and physical activity.

A first line of therapeutic intervention for individuals with MetS is regular physical activity, consumption of a heart healthy diet, weight loss (if necessary), and prevention of weight gain after weight loss. All five of the components that define MetS can be mitigated when these lifestyle behaviors are consistently practiced [42,43]. Of course, additional efforts should be made to quit smoking, improve stress management, and practice other appropriate behavioral techniques which increase the likelihood of long-term adherence to lifestyle changes (see also Chapter 7).

Adopting a healthy diet is of critical importance in terms of treating and managing components of MetS [44,45]. A variety of healthy diets are available which are very consistent with each other. This includes a Mediterranean-style diet composed of whole grain foods, fruit, vegetables, fish, fiber, and nuts which has been clearly demonstrated to lower CVD risk. Individuals who consume moderate amounts of alcohol as a component of the Mediterranean diet lower the risk of CVD and T2DM. The evidence-based dietary recommendations from AHA, NCEP-ATP III, and DASH diet [46] are also widely used in clinical practice and consistent with the recommendations of the Mediterranean diet [47]. All these diets would be considered plant-based diets and are the ones recommended by the Dietary Guidelines for Americans (DGA) 2020–2025 [48].

Physical activity recommendations are also quite consistent across multiple organizations and have been recently summarized by the Physical Activity Guidelines for Americans 2018 [49]. These guidelines recommend that individuals engage in 150 minutes of moderate physical activity on a weekly basis. The health benefits of regularly practiced physical activity occur in virtually every metabolic disease.

Weight loss is a top priority in patients with obesity who have MetS. The current recommendation is to achieve a 5%–10% reduction of body weight over 6–12 months through caloric restriction and increased physical activity [50,51]. The most efficacious weight loss programs include both regular physical activity and reduction in energy intake. Weight loss achieved by these healthy lifestyle behaviors may be the most effective way of preventing and treating MetS.

Other components of MetS including dyslipidemia, elevated blood pressure, and blood glucose management are all consistent with those for the prevention and treatment of CVD and T2DM and are discussed in detail in Chapters 12 and 13.

Weight loss is also an effective treatment for reducing inflammation.

14.9   SUMMARY/CONCLUSIONS

Obesity represents a worldwide pandemic. While not all individuals with obesity will develop metabolic complications, there is clearly an association between obesity and insulin resistance and chronic hyperinsulinemia which are primary factors that precipitate the clinical manifestations of MetS and increase CVD risk.

There are also considerable data to support the contribution of ectopic fat distribution in the high prevalence of MetS among overweight and obese individuals.

Clinicians should be well versed in recommendations for introducing therapeutic lifestyle changes to all patients but, in particular, to patients who are overweight and obese. Lifestyle modifications for individuals with obesity who have MetS should include weight loss, healthy nutrition, and regular physical activity. High-risk individuals may require pharmacologic interventions to complement lifestyle changes.

CLINICAL APPLICATIONS

- Clinicians should be aware of the diagnostic criteria from NCEP-ATP-III for MetS.
- All patients who are overweight or obese should be evaluated for potential MetS.
- While not all individuals with obesity have MetS, it is more prevalent in individuals who are overweight or obese than healthy weight individuals.
- The diagnosis of MetS can help with counseling individuals to lower their risk of both CVD and T2DM.

REFERENCES

1. Kylin E. Studien uber das Hypertonie-Hyperglykamie-Hyperurikamiesyndrom. *Zentralblatt fur Innere Medizin*. 1923;44:105–127.
2. Reaven G. Banting Lecture 1988. Role of insulin resistance in human disease. *Diabetes*. 1988;37:1595–1607.
3. Ford E. Increasing prevalence of the metabolic syndrome among U.S. adults. *Diabetes Care*. 2004;27:2444–2449.
4. Ford E., Giles W., Dietz W. Prevalence of the metabolic syndrome among U.S. adults. Findings from the third National Health and Nutrition Examination Survey. *JAMA*. 2002;287:356–359.
5. Ford E. Prevalence of the metabolic syndrome defined by the international diabetes federation among adults in the U.S. *Diabetes Care*. 2005;28:2745–2749.
6. Ford E., Zhao G. Prevalence and correlates of metabolic syndrome based on a harmonious definition among adults in the U.S. *J Diabetes*. 2010;3:180–193.
7. Flegal K., Carroll M., Ogden C., et al. Prevalence and trends in obesity among US adults, 1999–2008. *JAMA*. 2010;303:235–241.
8. Rasouli N., Molavi B., Elbien S., et al. Ectopic fat accumulation and metabolic syndrome. *Diabetes Obes Metab*. 2007;9:1–10.
9. Koh K., Han S., Quon M. Inflammatory markers and the metabolic syndrome. Insights from therapeutic interventions. *J Am Coll Cardiol*. 2005;46:1978–1985.
10. National Cholesterol Education Program. Executive Summary of the Third Report of the National Cholesterol Education Program (NCEP) Expert Panel on Detection, Evaluation and Treatment of High Blood Cholesterol in Adults (Adult Treatment Panel III). *JAMA*. 2001;285:2486–2497.
11. Alberti K., Eckel R., Grundy S., et al. Harmonizing the metabolic syndrome. A joint interim statement of the international diabetes federation task force on epidemiology and prevention; National Heart, Lung, Blood Institute; American Heart Association; World Heart Federation; International Atherosclerosis Society; and International Association for the Study of Obesity. *Circulation*. 2009;120:1640–1645.

12. Alberti K., Zimmet P., Shaw J. Metabolic syndrome - a new worldwide definition. A consensus statement from the International Diabetes Federation. *Diabet Med.* 2006;23:469–480.
13. Dunstan D., Zimmet P., Welborne T., et al. The rising prevalence of diabetes and impaired glucose tolerance. The Australian diabetes, obesity and lifestyle study. *Diabetes Care.* 2002;25:829–834.
14. Flegal K., Carroll M., Ogden C., et al. Prevalence and trends in obesity among US adults, 1999–2000. *JAMA.* 2002;288:1723–1727.
15. Hedley A., Ogden C., Johnson C., et al. Prevalence of overweight and obesity among US children, adolescents, and adults, 1999–2002. *JAMA.* 2004;291:2847–2850.
16. Park Y., Zhu S., Palaniappan L., et al. The metabolic syndrome: prevalence and associated risk factor findings in the U.S. population from the third National Health and Nutrition Examination Survey, 1988–1994. *Arch Intern Med.* 2003;163:427–436.
17. Stefan N., Kantartzis K., Machann J., et al. Identification and characterization of metabolically benign obesity in humans. *Arch Intern Med.* 2008;168:1609–1616.
18. Kim S., Reaven G. The metabolic syndrome: One step forward, two steps back. *Diabetes Vasc Dis Res.* 2004;2:68–75.
19. McLaughlin T., Allison G., Abbasi F., et al. Prevalence of insulin resistance and associated cardiovascular disease risk factors among normal weight, overweight, and obese individuals. *Metabolism.* 2004;53:495–499.
20. Stolar M. Metabolic syndrome: Controversial but useful. *Cleve Clin J Med.* 2007;74:199–208.
21. Wildman R., Munter P., Reynolds K., et al. The obese without cardiometabolic risk factor clustering and the normal weight with cardiometabolic risk factor clustering. *Arch Intern Med.* 2008;168:1617–1624.
22. Mottillo S., Filion K., Genest J., et al. The metabolic syndrome and cardiovascular risk. *J Am Coll Cardiol.* 2010;56:1113–1132.
23. Gami A., Witt B., Howard D., et al. Metabolic syndrome and risk of incident cardiovascular events and death. *J Am Coll Cardiol.* 2007;49:403–414.
24. Ford E., Li C., Sattar N. Metabolic syndrome and incident diabetes. *Diabetes Care.* 2008;31:1898–1904.
25. Wilson P., D'Agostino R., Parise H., et al. Metabolic syndrome as a precursor of cardiovascular disease and type 2 diabetes mellitus. *Circulation.* 2005;112:3066–3072.
26. Lakka H., Laaksonen D., Lakka T., et al. The metabolic syndrome and total and cardiovascular disease mortality in middle-aged men. *JAMA.* 2002;288:2709–2716.
27. Kurl S., Laukkanen J., Niskanen L., et al. Metabolic syndrome and the risk of stroke in middle-aged men. *Stroke.* 2006;37:806–811.
28. Le Roith D., Zick Y. Recent advances in our understanding of insulin action and insulin resistance. *Diabetes Care.* 2001;24:588–597.
29. Cusi K., Maezono K., Osman A., et al. Insulin resistance differentially affects the PI-3 kinase- and MAP-kinase-mediated signaling in human muscle. *J Clin Invest.* 2000;105:311–320.
30. DeFronzo R. Pathogenesis of type 2 diabetes mellitus. *Med Clin North Am.* 2004;88:787–835.
31. Lakka T., Lakka H., Salonen R., et al. Abdominal obesity is associated with accelerated progression of carotid atherosclerosis in men. *Atherosclerosis.* 2001;154:497–504.
32. Kenchaiah S., Evans J., Levy D., et al. Obesity and the risk of heart failure. *N Engl J Med.* 2002;347:305–313.
33. Despres J., Lemieux I. Abdominal obesity and metabolic syndrome. *Nature.* 2006;444:881–887.
34. Despres J. Cardiovascular disease under the influence of excess visceral fat. *Crit Pathways Cardiol.* 2007;6:51–59.

35. Eckhardt K., Taube A., Eckel J. Obesity-associated insulin resistance in skeletal muscle: Role of lipid accumulation and physical inactivity. *Rev Endocr Metab Disord.* 2011;12:163. E-pub ahead of print.
36. Meijer R., Serne E., Smulders Y., et al. Perivascular adipose tissue and its role in type 2 diabetes and cardiovascular disease. *Curr Diab Rep.* 2011;11:211–217.
37. Aguilera C., Gil-Campos M., Canete R., et al. Alterations in plasma and tissue lipids associated with obesity and metabolic syndrome. *Clin Sci.* 2008;114:183–193.
38. Adiels M., Taskinen M., Packard C., et al. Overproduction of VLDL particles is driven by increased liver fat content in man. *Diabetologia.* 2006;49:755–765.
39. Seppala-Lindroos A., Vehkavaara S., Hakkinen A., et al. Fat accumulation in the liver is associated with defects in insulin suppression of glucose production and serum free fatty acids independent of obesity in normal men. *J Clin Endocrinol Metab.* 2002;87:3023–3028.
40. Balkau B., Qiao Q., Tuomilehto J., Borch-Johnsen K., et al. Does the metabolic syndrome detect further subjects at high risk of cardiovascular death, or is a cardiovascular risk score adequate? *Diabetologia.* 2005;48:315.
41. Tota-Maharaj R., Defilipps A., Blumenthal R., et al. A practical approach to the metabolic syndrome: review of current concepts and management. *Curr Opin Clin Cardiol.* 2010;25:502–512.
42. Zhu S., St-Onge M., Heshka S., et al. Lifestyle behaviors associated with lower risk of having the metabolic syndrome. *Metabolism.* 2004;53:1503–1511.
43. Ratner R., Goldberg R., Haffner S., et al. Impact of intensive lifestyle and metformin therapy on cardiovascular disease risk factors in the Diabetes Prevention Program. *Diabetes Care.* 2005;28:888–894.
44. Blaha M., Bansal S., Rouf R., et al. A practical "ABCDE" approach to the metabolic syndrome. *Mayo Clin Proc.* 2008;83:932–943.
45. Grundy S., Cleeman J., Daniels S., et al. Diagnosis and management of the metabolic syndrome. An American Heart Association/National Heart, Lung, and Blood Institute Scientific Statement. *Circulation.* 2005;112:2735–2752.
46. The DASH Diet Eating Plan. http://dashdiet.org/default.asp. Accessed August 25, 2020.
47. Shai I., Schwarzfuchs D., Henkin Y., et al. Weight loss with a low-carbohydrate, Mediterranean, or low-fat diet. *N Engl J Med.* 2008;359:229–241.
48. U.S. Department of Agriculture and U.S. Department of Health and Human Services. Dietary Guidelines for Americans, 2020–2025. 9th Edition. December 2020. Available at DietaryGuidelines.gov. Accessed January 19, 2021.
49. 2018 Physical Activity Guidelines Advisory Committee. 2018 Physical Activity Guidelines Advisory Committee Scientific Report. Washington, DC: U.S. Department of Health and Human Services, 2018.
50. National Institutes of Health. Clinical guidelines on the identification, evaluation, and treatment of overweight and obese adults - the evidence report. National Institutes of Health. *Obesity Res.* 1998;6:51S–209S.
51. Donnelly J., Blair S., Jakicic J., et al. Appropriate physical activity intervention strategies for weight loss and prevention of weight regain for adults. *Med Sci Sports Exer.* 2009;41:459–471.

15 Lifestyle Approaches Targeting Obesity to Lower Cancer Risk, Progression, and Recurrence

James M. Rippe, MD
Rippe Lifestyle Institute
University of Massachusetts Medical School

CONTENTS

15.1 INTRODUCTION

Obesity is a major health problem in the United States. It represents one of the major public health challenges of our time [1,2]. On a global basis, obesity has reached pandemic proportions affecting an estimated 2.1 billion adults with obesity and 110 million children with obesity [3,4]. Obesity is well-known to increase the risk of various metabolic diseases including cardiovascular disease (CVD) and type 2 diabetes (T2DM). Few clinicians and the public at large realize that individuals with obesity or who are overweight also carry an increased risk and worse prognosis of multiple malignancies [5].

Of note, in 1962 only 14.3% of the US adult population was estimated to be with obesity [6]. More recent US data indicate that the prevalence of obesity is 42.5% of adults with higher rates in adult women and slightly lower rates in men [7].

DOI: 10.1201/9781003099116-17

While the public is generally aware of the impact of obesity on CVD and T2DM, the impact of overweight and obesity cancer is much less well known. In fact, in 2017 a report from the American Institute of Cancer Research (AICR) indicated that only 50% of Americans were aware that obesity stimulates cancer growth [8].

The International Agency for Cancer Research (IACR) extensively reviewed epidemiologic data and concluded that 13 human malignancies are linked to excess body fatness [9]. These include gastrointestinal tract tumors (e.g. esophageal adenocarcinoma), gastric cardia cancer, rectal cancer, liver cancer, gall bladder, and pancreatic cancer. Obesity is also linked to other malignancies including post-menopausal breast cancer; ovarian, renal cell, and thyroid cancers; meningioma and multiple myeloma. There are also suggestive, but not conclusive, data that some other malignancies including hematologic malignancies, prostate cancer, and even possibly lung cancer may be associated with obesity.

15.2   MECHANISMS OF OBESITY IMPACT ON CANCER

Adipose tissue was once considered to be a relatively passive storage depot where excess energy was maintained in the form of fats (triglycerides). However, it has now been shown that adipose tissue, which is composed of multiple cell types including adipocytes, stromal fibroblasts, and vascular immune and hematopoietic cells, is intensely metabolic with multiple physiologic functions including inflammation, modulation of insulin sensitivity, appetite regulation, nutrient uptake and storage, and many other physiologic processes. These multiple effects of adipose tissue create pathophysiologic mechanisms through which obesity promotes cancer.

Multiple effects of adipose tissue result in alterations in metabolic, hormonal, and pro-inflammatory signals and pathways which have an impact on cancer. It is important to note that obesity is not considered to be the initiating factor for the carcinogenic process but rather promotes cancer progression [10]. Multiple mechanisms have been postulated for this association. As adipose tissue expands, adipose cells expand and enlarge and some undergo cell death (apoptosis) which underscores an inflammatory process and yields increased inflammatory factors such as cytokines, lipids, IL-6, IL-1, and TNF-α [11,12]. These, in turn, create an environment which creates or can lead to insulin resistance as well as stimulating increases in leptin and, in turn, downregulates adiponectin which has an appetite-stimulating function [13].

Levels of insulin and insulin-like growth factor (IGF-1) typically increase in obesity and may contribute to tumor growth. Elevated levels of insulin promote tumor cell growth and cancer progression. IGF-1 can also contribute to tumor cell growth. Aromatase which is an enzyme responsible for converting androstenedione to estrone and estrogen is found at increased levels in obesity yielding increased estrogen which, in turn, promotes the growth of breast cancer.

In addition, the intestinal microbiome in overweight and obesity may further increase the risk of cancer. It has also been demonstrated that fat cells may take up and metabolize cancer chemotherapeutic agents and thereby reduce available chemotherapy in the tumor microenvironment [14]. Obesity may also alter the genetic processes that result in altered proteins in ways that promote cancer growth.

It should also be noted that not all adipose tissue has the same metabolic hormonal or pro-inflammatory activity. Visceral fat, for example, which is fat found in or around abdominal organs, is more intensely metabolic and pro-inflammatory than subcutaneous fat [15–17]. In epidemiologic studies, visceral fat has been linked to tumor promotion in humans.

Weight loss and calorie constriction can decrease both visceral and subcutaneous fat [18]. A variety of pharmacologic interventions which block insulin or IGF receptors may also positively affect a reduction in breast cancer.

In addition to obesity itself, various dietary fats may have an impact on cancer. In general, tumor-promoting fatty acids such as medium-chain saturated fatty acids such as lauric and myristic as well as long-chained fatty acids including palmitic and stearic acid may promote cancer growth [19]. Unsaturated fats such as oleic and polyunsaturated fats have anti-inflammatory properties and can function as tumor suppressors [20,21].

High carbohydrate diets that result in hyperglycemia and insulin resistance in individuals with obesity or with diabetes have also been shown in some models to potentially contribute to cancer progression [22,23]. For example, in patients with Stage 3 colon cancer and elevated BMI who failed chemotherapy, increased glycemic and carbohydrate loads led to shorter overall survival [24].

15.3 STRATEGIES TO DISRUPT THE OBESITY/CANCER LINKAGE

Clearly the most effective way to prevent increased cancer risk associated with obesity to maintain a lean body mass throughout life utilizing the established lifestyle practices of dietary regulation and regular physical activity.

For individuals who are overweight or obese, weight loss is the most effective way of reducing the risk of cancer [25–27]. Studies in patients with obesity have demonstrated that weight loss can lower various inflammatory markers as well as insulin and IGF-1. This benefit only occurs for sustained weight loss. Changes in dietary composition have only been shown to be effective in the primary prevention of breast cancer when they are accompanied by weight loss. Reduced fats diets also may result in risk reduction when coupled with weight loss in post-menopausal women with hormone receptor negative tumors.

The most convincing beneficial consequences of intentional weight loss have been demonstrated in bariatric surgery. For example, the Swedish Obesity Subjects (SOS) prospective study which compared outcomes in over 2,000 surgery patients to a similar number of controls showed a 40% reduction in cancer incidence after 10.9 years of follow-up. Even greater reductions in cancer were shown in a study from Utah of 7,925 patients compared to 7,955 controls which showed a 60% decrease in cancer mortality following bariatric surgery.

Taken as a whole, this literature suggests that significant and sustained weight loss and restoration of lean body mass is required to reduce cancer incidence among patients with obesity or who are overweight. However, it should be emphasized that maintaining a lean body mass throughout life by adopting lifestyle practices such as attention to sound nutrition and regular physical activity provides the best outcomes with regard to reducing cancer risk.

15.4 LIFESTYLE RECOMMENDATIONS TO DISRUPT THE OBESITY/CANCER LINKAGE

- *Recommendations for lifestyle modifications for primary cancer prevention*: As already indicated, maintaining a healthy BMI (18.5–24.9 kg/m^2) throughout life is important to prevent many common types of cancers. While numerous guidelines suggest what constitutes a healthy approach to weight management, they consistently focus on diet and physical activity. A number of guidelines for physical activity and diet for cancer prevention are available and are outlined in Table 15.1.

  Good evidence exists in a variety of lifestyle-related habits and practices which will be discussed in the next few sections of this chapter.
- *Achieve and maintain lean weight across the life span*: A body mass index between 18.5 and 24.9 kg/m^2 is considered a healthy weight and is associated with decreased risk for developing many metabolic diseases such as T2DM, hypertension, coronary heart disease (CHD), stroke, and many cancers. Increased weight at any time of life may result in obesity at later stages and may also have long-lasting epigenetic effects. For example, adult weight gain is significantly associated with an increased risk of post-menopausal breast cancer [28], endometrial and ovarian cancers, and colon cancers in men. Long-term weight management and participation in regular physical activity and attention to nutrition practices are all important in terms of maintaining long-term maintenance of a healthy weight.
- *Avoid high-calorie foods*: A major contributor to the obesity epidemic is the availability and appeal of energy-dense foods [29]. This includes foods that are high in fat, energy-dense drinks such as sugary ones containing large amounts of sugar which should be minimized as should be fast foods.
- *Prioritize healthy eating patterns*: Because vegetables and fruits as well as legumes and whole grains are high in fiber and water and low in fat, they represent perfect examples of low energy-dense foods that promote both

---

TABLE 15.1
Obesity Cancer Guidelines

American Cancer Society Guidelines for Diet and Physical Activity	https://www.cancer.org/healthy/eat-healthy-get-active/-acs-guidelines-nutrition-physical-activity-cancer-prevention.html
American Institute for Cancer Research – Cancer Prevention Recommendation	https://www.aicr.org/cancer-prevention/
National Heart, Lung and Blood Institute	https://www.nhlbi.nih.gov/
US Department of Health and Human Services: President's Council on Sports, Fitness & Nutrition	https://www.hhs.gov/fitness/index.html

maintenance lean healthy weight as well as representing key components of weight loss [30] (see also Chapter 6 on nutritional strategies in cancer).

- *Physical activity*: Physical activity carries many health benefits. Physical activity can result in increased caloric expenditure and also enhance maintenance or increase of lean muscle mass [31]. Regular physical activity is a key for the maintenance of a healthy weight and also lowers the risk of weight gain and obesity (See also Chapter 5).
- *Maintain good sleep hygiene*: Sleep is an important component of weight management. This appears to be a function of a variety of biological mechanisms which regulate hormonal rhythms [32]. Inadequate sleep has been associated with many diseases, including obesity. In addition, lack of adequate sleep can increase the risk of both heart disease and diabetes (See also Chapters 12 and 13).
- *Lose weight if you have obesity or are overweight*: Weight loss either through a weight management program or bariatric surgery has been shown to play a significant role in the primary prevention of cancer [33]. More detail on these programs is found in Chapters 7 and 9.
- *Follow cancer screening protocols*: For individuals with obesity or who are overweight, there is often a tendency to avoid cancer screening. It is, however, important to remember that obesity increases the risk of cancer occurrence and that early detection increases the chance of cure and decreases the need for more extensive therapies. For all of these reasons, it is important that individuals with obesity or who are overweight follow the recommended cancer screening guidelines for breast, color rectal, lung, and gynecologic cancers [34–37].
- *Guidelines for secondary prevention in cancer survivors*: Guidelines for secondary prevention in cancer survivors are quite similar to those in primary prevention of cancer. Cancer survivorship is, of course, life after the diagnosis of cancer. The goal after a diagnosis is either a cure or lengthening survival and decreasing complications related to therapy as well as preventing or detecting new primary cancers.

   The number of cancer survivors has increased substantially in the past decades. Currently, there are more than 15.5 million cancer survivors in the US [38]. These individuals face substantial challenges not only in recovering but living with consequences of their diagnosis and treatment. It may also be more difficult for these individuals to maintain healthy lifestyle modifications that can lead to improved health outcomes.
- *Avoid weight gain following cancer diagnosis*: Obesity is a risk factor for cancer occurrence after the initial diagnosis and treatment and can lead to worse outcomes [39–41]. Obese cancer survivors are more likely to develop complications from cancer treatment. Therefore, following an initial cancer diagnosis, obesity should be aggressively treated as a risk factor which needs to be controlled just as tobacco use does [42–44].

   Many interventions aiming to control cancer can also lead to the adverse consequences of weight gain. These include medications to prevent nausea and reactions to chemotherapy as well as the development of fatigue as a cancer symptom or side effect. Furthermore, the development of side effects such as neuropathy, myalgia, and arthralgia can make regular forms of exercise more difficult and challenging. The use of hormonal manipulation (e.g. in breast or prostate cancer) can result in decreased muscle mass. Gastrointestinal side effects, such as changes in taste, nausea, diarrhea, and constipation, can lead to the decreased likelihood of nutritious food choices and may skew food intake toward unhealthy food groups.

Finally, sleep dysfunction, which is a common manifestation of cancer side effects from treatment and as already discussed, can contribute to weight gain.

Recommendations both for primary prevention of cancer as well as secondary prevention in cancer survivors are summarized in Table 15.2

- *The role of exercise to decrease obesity*: Different forms of exercise have been demonstrated to be effective to combat the side effects of treatment [45,46]. Both aerobic and resistance training exercises can improve cancer-related fatigue. The biological reasons for the protective effects of exercise may be more complex simply than weight management. For example, exercise can modulate circulating levels of both insulin and IGF-1 [47,48]. The role of physical activity in reducing the risk of cancer is outlined in more detail in Chapter 5.

- *Nutritional changes to achieve weight loss*: Dietary interventions may also be helpful as a form of secondary cancer prevention. For example, the consumption of fruits and vegetables and decreased consumption of dietary fat may lead to weight loss. In the Women's Initiative in Nutrition Study (WINS), analysis found a 24% lower risk of breast cancer recurrence and a 42% lower recurrence risk in hormonal receptor negative breast cancer patients [49]. It should be noted that this may be partially a result of the weight loss that was experienced in the intervention group. These individuals lost an average of six pounds.

- *Sleep hygiene*: Just as in primary prevention of cancer good sleep hygiene is important in cancer survivors. This is particularly true because many cancer survivors suffer from sleep disruption such as insomnia which can be a result either from concern about the diagnosis or side effects from its treatment.

15.5   TYPE 2 DIABETES MELLITUS AND CANCER RISK

There is a strong correlation between obesity and the development of T2DM (see also Chapter 13). T2DM is a condition that is defined by insulin resistance leading to sustained hyperinsulinemia and hyperglycemia. T2DM is associated with an increased risk for a variety of malignancies including pancreatic, colon, endometrial, breast, and hepatobiliary cancers [50–52]. One hypothesis for the increased cancer risk seen in T2DM is the cancer-promoting effect of insulin and IGF-1, the levels of which are typically elevated in this population. T2DM is associated with excess mortality in multiple cancer types including colorectal, breast, pancreatic, gastric, liver, endometrial, and even lung cancers.

There are some data that suggest that one of the therapies for T2DM, such as Metformin, has antineoplastic effects [53]. There is controversy concerning

TABLE 15.2
Recommendations for Lifestyle Modifications for Primary Cancer Prevention

Achieve and maintain a lean weight across life span	Healthy BMI for adults: 18.5–24.9 Adolescents and children over age 2: BMI between 5th and 85th percentile for the age
If overweight or obese, lose weight gradually	Weight loss goal: 1–2 pounds per week
Avoid calorie-dense foods and sugary drinks	Drink more water and avoid high glycemic foods such as desserts, sodas, white breads
Prioritize healthy eating patterns, eating plant-based whole foods that are not calorie dense but nutrient dense (high in vitamins and minerals) and high in fiber content	Consume at least five portions of vegetables and fruits of different colors (dark leafy greens, orange, red, yellow, and purple) daily. Use legumes (beans) as a major source of protein.
Limit the amount of certain animal-derived foods	Red meat (beef, pork, lamb, goat) should be limited to <500 g/week. If consuming animal protein, prioritize fish and poultry
Consider adopting a well-balanced vegetarian or vegan (whole foods, completely plant-based) diet	Whole foods, plant-based diet aid in weight loss and maintenance of healthy weight through avoidance of calorie-dense foods while providing ample amounts of protein, minerals, and vitamins
Engage in physical exercise	Aim for at least 150 minutes of moderate exercise (brisk walk, biking, yoga) or 75 minutes of vigorous exercise (swimming, running/jogging) per week
Avoid completely the use of tobacco and if drinking alcohol, use moderation	Men should limit alcohol intake to up to 2 drinks per day and women to less than 1 drink per day. One standard drink = 5 oz glass of wine, 1.5 oz hard liquor, 12 oz beer. Alcohol is a calorie-dense drink and can lead to weight gain.
Prioritize sleep	Aim for 7–8 hours of sleep every night
Avoid dietary supplements unless prescribed by a physician	Obtain all vitamins and minerals from your diet. People following a strict plant-based diet (vegan diet) require oral B12 supplementation
If unable to lose weight by making all aforementioned recommendations, consider joining a weight management program	Achieving and keeping a healthy BMI should be a priority. Discuss with primary care provider bariatric surgery evaluation if behavior modifications fail to promote meaningful weight loss

Bruno D., Berger N. Lifestyle Approaches Targeting Obesity to Reduce Cancer Risk, Progress & Recurrence. Reprinted from *Obesity Prevention and Treatment* by Rippe J.M. and Angelopoulos, T.J. CRC Press (Boca Raton), 2012. Used with permission of the editor Dr. James Rippe.

whether or not there is an association with insulin use in T2DM and increased risk of cancer [54].

15.6　CONCLUSIONS

Obesity is a substantial risk factor for many malignancies. Excessive adipose tissue can promote tumor progression through a variety of mechanisms, including inflammatory, hormonal, and epigenetic alterations. Therefore, maintaining a healthy body weight across the lifespan is an excellent practice for cancer prevention and secondary treatment.

CLINICAL APPLICATIONS

- All patients with obesity or who are overweight should be counseled about the importance of weight loss.
- Individuals who are within the healthy weight range (BMI 18.5–24.9) should be counseled concerning the link between adult weight gain and overweight or obesity and cancer.
- Lifestyle measures such as attention to nutritious and calorie-controlled diet as well as physical activity are both recognized and important modalities for reducing the risk of cancer and assisting in the long-term survival of cancer survivors.

REFERENCES

1. Bassett M., Perl S. Obesity: The public health challenge of our time. *Am J Public Health.* 2004;94(9):1477.
2. Hurt R., Kulisek C., Buchanan L.A., et al. The obesity epidemic: Challenges, health initiatives, and implications for gastroenterologists. *Gastroenterol Hepatol.* 2010;6(12):780–92.
3. Ezzati M. Trends in adult body mass index in 200 countries from 1975 to 2014: A pooled analysis of 1698 population-based measurement studies with 19.2 million participants. *Lancet.* 2016;387(10026):1377–96.
4. Afshin A., Forouzanfar M., Reitsma M., et al. Health effects of overweight and obesity in 195 countries over 25 years. *N Engl J Med.* 2017;377(1):13–27.
5. Massetti G., Dietz W., Richardson L. Excessive weight gain, obesity, and cancer: opportunities for clinical intervention. *JAMA.* 2017;318:1975–6.
6. Ogden C., Carroll M. Prevalence of overweight, obesity, and extreme obesity among adults: united states, trends 1960–1962 through 2007–2008: NCHS - Health E-Stats, 2010; https://www.cdc.gov/nchs/data/hestat/overweight/overweight.htm. Accessed on August 27, 2020.
7. Fryar C., Carroll M., Ogden C.L. CDC: National Center for Health Statistics. Prevalence of Overweight, Obesity, and Severe Obesity among Children and Adolescents Aged 2–19 Years: United States, 1963–1965 Through 2015–2016. Division of Health and Nutrition Examination Surveys. https://www.cdc.gov/nchs/data/hestat/obesity_child_15_16/obesity_child_15_16.pdf. Accessed on January 2021.
8. American Institute for Cancer Research. Cancer Risk Awareness Infographic 2017. https://www.aicr.org/news/survey-finds-alarming-gaps-in-americans-knowledge-of-major-cancer-risk-factors/#:~:text=The%20AICR%20survey%20finds%20that, Americans%20have%20overweight%20or%20obesity. Accessed on August 27, 2020.

9. Lauby-Secretan B., Scoccianti C., Loomis D., et al. Body fatness and cancer—Viewpoint of the IARC working group. *N Engl J Med.* 2016;375(8):794–8.

10. Berger N. Obesity and cancer pathogenesis. *Ann N Y Acad Sci.* 2014;1311:57–76.

11. Hotamisligil G. Inflammation and metabolic disorders. *Nature.* 2006;444(7121):860–7.

12. Reilly S., Saltiel A. Adapting to obesity with adipose tissue inflammation. *Nat Rev Endocrin.* 2017;13(11):633–43.

13. O'Leary V., Kirwan J. Adiponectin, obesity, and cancer. In: Reizes O. Berger N.A., editors. *Adipocytokines, Energy Balance, and Cancer.* Cham: Springer International Publishing; 2017, pp. 21–38.

14. Sheng X., Parmentier J., Tucci J., et al. Adipocytes sequester and metabolize the chemotherapeutic daunorubicin. *Mol Cancer Res.* 2017;15(12):1704–13.

15. Qiang G., Kong H., Fang D., et al. The obesity-induced transcriptional regulator TRIP-Br2 mediates visceral fat endoplasmic reticulum stress-induced inflammation. *Nat Commun.* 2016;7:11378.

16. Lee M., Wu Y., Fried S. Adipose tissue heterogeneity: Implication of depot differences in adipose tissue for obesity complications. *Mol Aspects Med.* 2013;34(1):1–11.

17. Tchkonia T., Thomou T., Zhu Y., et al. Mechanisms and metabolic implications of regional differences among fat depots. *Cell Metab.* 2013;17(5):644–56.

18. Hill-Baskin A., Markiewski M., Buchner D., et al. Diet-induced hepatocellular carcinoma in genetically predisposed mice. *Hum Mol Genet.* 2009;18(16):2975–88.

19. Doerner S., Reis E., Leung E., et al. High-fat diet-induced complement activation mediates intestinal inflammation and neoplasia, independent of obesity. *Mol Cancer Res.* 2016;14(10):953–65.

20. Iyengar N., Hudis C., Gucalp A. Omega-3 fatty acids for the prevention of breast cancer: An update and state of the science. *Curr Breast Cancer Rep.* 2013;5(3):247–54.

21. Azrad M., Turgeon C., Demark- Wahnefried W. Current evidence linking polyunsaturated Fatty acids with cancer risk and progression. *Front Oncol.* 2013;3:224.

22. Healy M., Lahiri S., Hargett S., et al. Dietary sugar intake increases liver tumor incidence in female mice. *Sci Rep.* 2016;6:22292.

23. Thompson C., Khiani V., Chak A., et al. Carbohydrate consumption and esophageal cancer: An ecological assessment. *Am J Gastroenterol.* 2008;103(3):555–61.

24. Meyerhardt J., Sato K., Niedzwiecki D., et al. Dietary glycemic load and cancer recurrence and survival in patients with stage III colon cancer: Findings from CALGB 89803. *J Natl Cancer Inst.* 2012;104(22):1702–11.

25. Linkov F., Maxwell G., Felix A.S., et al. Longitudinal evaluation of cancer associated biomarkers before and after weight loss in RENEW study participants: Implications for cancer risk reduction. *Gynecol Oncol.* 2012;125(1):114–9.

26. Parker E., Folsom A. Intentional weight loss and incidence of obesity related cancers: The Iowa Women's Health Study. *Int J Obes Rel Metab Disord: J Int Assoc Study Obes.* 2003;27(12):1447–52.

27. Byers T., Sedjo R. Does intentional weight loss reduce cancer risk? *Diabetes Obes Metab.* 2011;13(12):1063–72.

28. Keum N., Greenwood D., Lee D., et al. Adult weight gain and adiposity-related cancers: A dose-response meta-analysis of prospective observational studies. *J Natl Cancer Inst.* 2015;107(2):djv088.

29. Hendrickson K. How to Calculate Energy from Foods Livestrong.com 2017. https://www.livestrong.com/article/312047-how-to-calculate-energy-from-foods/. Accessed on August 27, 2020.

30. CDC. Low-Energy-Dense Foods and Weight Management: Cutting Calories While Controlling Hunger. https://www.cdc.gov/healthyweight/healthy_eating/energy_density.html. Accessed on August 27, 2020.

31. 2018 Physical Activity Guidelines Advisory Committee. 2018 Physical Activity Guidelines Advisory Committee Scientific Report. Washington, DC: U.S. Department of Health and Human Services, 2018.

32. Taheri S., Lin L., Austin D., et al. Short sleep duration is associated with reduced leptin, elevated ghrelin, and increased body mass index. *PLoS Med.* 2004;1(3):e62.

33. Kushner R., Ryan D. Assessment and lifestyle management of patients with obesity: Clinical recommendations from systematic reviews. *JAMA.* 2014;312(9):943–52.

34. Oeffinger K., Fontham E., Etzioni R., et al. Breast cancer screening for women at average risk: 2015 guideline update from the American Cancer Society. *JAMA.* 2015;314(15):1599–614.

35. Siu A. Screening for breast cancer: U.S. Preventive services task force recommendation statement. *Ann Intern Med.* 2016;164(4):279–96.

36. Lin J., Piper M., Perdue L., et al. Screening for colorectal cancer: Updated evidence report and systematic review for the US preventive services task force. *JAMA.* 2016;315(23):2576–94.

37. Saslow D., Solomon D., Lawson H., et al. American Cancer Society, American Society for Colposcopy and Cervical Pathology, and American Society for Clinical

38. Pathology screening guidelines for the prevention and early detection of cervical cancer. *CA: Cancer J Clin.* 2012;62(3):147–72.

38. American Cancer Society. Cancer Facts and Figures 2017. Atlanta, GA: The American Cancer Society; 2017.

39. Chan D., Vieira A., Aune D., et al. Body mass index and survival in women with breast cancer-systematic literature review and meta-analysis of 82 follow-up studies. *Ann Oncol.* 2014;25(10):1901–14.

40. Meyerhardt J., Catalano P., Haller D.G. et al. Influence of body mass index on outcomes and treatment-related toxicity in patients with colon carcinoma. *Cancer.* 2003;98(3):484–95.

41. Efstathiou J., Bae K., Shipley W., et al. Obesity and mortality in men with locally advanced prostate cancer: Analysis of RTOG 85-31. *Cancer.* 2007;110(12):2691–9.

42. Paskett E., Dean J., Oliveri J., Harrop J.P. Cancer-related lymphedema risk factors, diagnosis, treatment, and impact: A review. *J Clin Oncol.* 2012;30(30):3726–33.

43. Meyerhardt J., Tepper J., Niedzwiecki D., et al. Impact of body mass index on outcomes and treatment-related toxicity in patients with stage II and III rectal cancer: Findings from Intergroup Trial 0114. *J Clin Oncol.* 2004;22(4):648–57.

44. Bouwman F., Smits A., Lopes A., et al. The impact of BMI on surgical complications and outcomes in endometrial cancer surgery–an institutional study and systematic review of the literature. *Gynecol Oncol.* 2015;139(2):369–76.

45. Mustian K., Sprod L., Janelsins M., et al. Exercise recommendations for cancer- related fatigue, cognitive impairment, sleep problems, depression, pain, anxiety, and physical dysfunction: A review. *Oncol Hematol Rev.* 2012;8(2):81–8.

46. Knols R., Aaronson N., Uebelhart D., et al. Physical exercise in cancer patients during and after medical treatment: A systematic review of randomized and controlled clinical trials. *J Clin Oncol.* 2005;23(16):3830–42.

47. Fairey A., Courneya K., Field C., et al. Effects of exercise training on fasting insulin, insulin resistance, insulin-like growth factors, and insulin-like growth factor binding proteins in postmenopausal breast cancer survivors: A randomized controlled trial. *Cancer Epidemiol Biomarkers Prev.* 2003;12(8):721–7.

48. Ligibel J., Campbell N., Partridge A., et al. Impact of a mixed strength and endurance exercise intervention on insulin levels in breast cancer survivors. *J Clin Oncol.* 2008;26(6):907–12.

49. Chlebowski R., Blackburn G., Thomson C., et al. Dietary fat reduction and breast cancer outcome: Interim efficacy results from the Women's Intervention Nutrition Study. *J Natl Cancer Inst.* 2006;98(24):1767–76.

50. Park S., Lim M., Shin S., et al. Impact of prediagnosis smoking, alcohol, obesity, and insulin resistance on survival in male cancer patients: National Health Insurance Corporation Study. *J Clin Oncol.* 2006;24(31):5017–24.

51. Barone B., Yeh H., Snyder C., et al. Long-term all-cause mortality in cancer patients with preexisting diabetes mellitus: A systematic review and meta-analysis. *JAMA.* 2008;300(23):2754–64.

52. Zhou G., Myers R., Li Y., et al. Role of AMP-activated protein kinase in mechanism of metformin action. *J Clin Invest.* 2001;108(8):1167–74.

53. Decensi A., Puntoni M., Goodwin P., et al. Metformin and cancer risk in diabetic patients: A systematic review and meta-analysis. *Cancer Prev Res.* 2010;3(11):1451–61.

54. Wu J., Azoulay L., Majdan A., et al. Long-term use of long-acting insulin analogs and breast cancer incidence in women with type 2 diabetes. *J Clin Oncol.* 2017;35(32):3647–53.

16 Obesity and Arthritis

James M. Rippe, MD
Rippe Lifestyle Institute
University of Massachusetts Medical School

CONTENTS

16.1 INTRODUCTION

Arthritis may affect any of the structures inside of joints including the synovium, bones, cartilage, and supporting tissues. As an inflammatory condition, arthritis gives rise to the classic signs of inflammation including pain, heat, redness, swelling, and, if left untreated, loss of function [1]. Inflammation is the normal response of the immune system to antigens [2]. Both osteoarthritis (the most common form of arthritis) and rheumatoid arthritis (the second most common form of arthritis) are common in the adult population. For example, osteoarthritis has a prevalence of greater than 10% in the general population and increases with age [3]. The exact causes of both osteoarthritis (OA) and rheumatoid arthritis (RA) are not completely known. It is clear, however, that both are associated to some degree with overweight or obesity.

16.2 OSTEOARTHRITIS

Osteoarthritis is by far the most common form of arthritis and one of the leading causes of pain and disability worldwide [4]. A variety of joint traumas may trigger the need for repair, but once initiated they often result in a chronic condition. Initially, there is an efficient repair process in OA. However, if the reason for the underlying arthritis is ongoing or overwhelming, eventually tissue damage occurs and eventually symptomatic OA ensues [5].

- *Potential causes of OA and the role of obesity*: There are multiple underlying conditions behind OA. These are generally divided into the categories of genetic, biomechanical, and constitutional factors [4].

DOI: 10.1201/9781003099116-18

Classic twin studies have shown that the role of genetic factors is between 39% and 65% for OA of the knee and about 60% for OA for the hip and 70% for OA in the spine. These percentages suggest a heritability of OA of more than 50%, suggesting that at least half of the variation in susceptibility to this disease can be explained by genetic factors alone [6].

Biomechanical risk factors and as in a previous joint injury, occupational and recreational usage, reduced muscle strength [7], joint laxity, or joint misalignment are commonly reported in OA patients. However, their validity of risk factors is not clear. Results from studies looking at occupational usage are not equivocal. For example, excessive kneeling, squatting, climbing steps, standing, and lifting may be associated with OA. Recreational exercise such as walking is not normally associated with OA. Conversely, in athletes and people who exercise excessively or intensively, OA is more common than in the general population.

Constitutional factors such a bone mineral density, age, gender, and body weight have also been implicated in the development and progression of OA [8,9]. Women have a higher instance of knee OA and are more than twice as likely as men to develop the condition [7]. The cause of this is not clear. The most possible explanation is that women actually have higher body fat reserves than men.

Obesity is the single strongest and most consistent constitutional risk factor for OA [10,11]. This has been supported by numerous studies over the last five decades. Overall, two-thirds of adults with physician diagnosed OA are overweight or obese, while greater than 30% of individuals with obesity suffer from OA compared to approximately 15% of non-obese adults. Women with OA have an average BMI about 24% higher than women without OA. Similarly, twins with OA are 3–5 kg heavier than their non-OA co-twin. For every kilogram increase in body weight a twin has a 9%, 14%, and 32% increased risk for developing carpometacarpal, tibiofemoral, and pattelofemoral osteophytes, respectively, compared to its co-twin.

- *Obesity and knee OA*: Knee OA shows the highest association with obesity. In one study, 83% of females diagnosed with OA of the knee were reported to have obesity (compared to 42% of the control group) [12]. A recent meta-analysis of 36 papers showed that overweight is more than twice as likely (OR 2.18) to lead to knee OA, while individuals with obesity are 2.63 times as likely compared to individuals of normal weight [2].

  The associations of obesity with knee OA seem to be independent of age or gender. They are, however, affected by the degree of obesity. For every two units of BMI gain, the risk of knee OA increases by 36% [13]. Individuals with a BMI > 40 kg/m^2 have almost a tenfold relative risk of OA development compared to normal-weight individuals [13]. Time of exposure (i.e. years of having obesity) is also important. Even small increases in body weight during adulthood increase the risk of developing OA. An estimated 69% of knee replacements in middle-aged women in the United Kingdom have been attributed to obesity [14].

- *Obesity and hand OA*: The site most commonly affected by OA is the small joints of the hand. In contrast to knee OA, data regarding the association of obesity with hand OA are conflicting [15]. Some studies have suggested that OA of the hand is more prevalent in individuals with obesity, but others have not found a significant association.
- *Obesity and hip OA*: Similarly to hand OA, the association of hip OA with obesity is not consistent. In the National Health and Nutrition Examination Survey (NHANES) study, weight was slightly associated with OA of the hips in white women and non-white men [16]. Longitudinal studies have not found any association between obesity and hip OA.
- *Mechanisms for obesity in the pathogenesis of OA*: The exact way by which obesity increases the risk of OA is not clear. Two potential mechanisms are most likely to play a significant role:
  1. Biomechanical factors from increased load on weight-bearing joints.
  2. Indirect systemic factors from the inflammatory nature of obesity.
     Biomechanical factors: Increasing body weight has a direct effect on vertical ground reaction forces (GRF). Simply by standing, males with obesity exert 53% more GRF, while females exert 45% more [17] than normal weight controls. During walking at normal speeds, the difference reaches up to 60% increase in GRF individuals with obesity. This has a particularly strong effect on plantar pressures which results in larger forefoot widths while standing and walking [18,19]. This commonly causes plantar fasciitis and heel pain which is also frequently present in older adults with OA.
     Even though it would be anticipated that individuals with obesity would be stronger than normal weight individuals, when strength is corrected for bodyweight both males and females with obesity are weaker compared to controls, irrespective of age. This relative muscular weakness is also a significant predictor of falls. Obesity further adds to such risks by affecting balance.
     In fact, the risk of injury increases with BMI. Fear of falls or other injuries is very likely an explanation for some of the observed changes in the gait of individuals with obesity. These individuals tend to walk with bilateral abducted forefeet (toes pointed outward) [20]. This appears to be a strategy to minimize the chance of falling but results in increased surface area, allowing for more sideways motion. This creates a variety of torques which further contribute to the development and progression of OA.
     Systemic factors: Low-grade inflammation is thought to be part of the process of obesity and may be implicated in the pathogenesis of OA [21]. OA patients exhibit increased levels of a variety of circulating inflammatory markers such as cytokines, interlukin-6 (IL-6), and tumor necrosis factor alpha (TNFα). High serum levels of these markers predict increased radiographic progression of knee OA as much as 5 years later. These problems are compounded in obesity which is increasingly being recognized as a low-grade inflammatory condition.

- *Effects of weight loss on OA*: Obesity is the most significant modifiable risk factor for the development and progression of OA. Maintaining a healthy body weight may prevent the development of OA. Reducing body weight in an OA patient may decelerate the process by diminishing forces applied to the joints as well as lowering systemic inflammatory loads. In the Framingham cohort, weight loss in mid or later life substantially reduced the risk of symptomatic OA of the knee [22]. A decrease in BMI of two units (approximate 5 kg on average) in the 10 years prior to assessment decreased the risk of OA development by 50%, irrespective of the initial BMI. The two most effective non-pharmacological treatments for increased body weight are diet and exercise.
- *Dietary interventions in OA*: Interventions which are aimed at reducing caloric intake with concomitant generation of energy deficits of 800–1,000 kcal/day with a minimum of 1,100–1,200 kcal remaining for men and women, respectively, are effective for weight loss [23]. A number of studies have demonstrated the efficacy of energy intake reduction. As with any weight loss intervention, the greatest challenge in weight loss is maintenance. The Arthritis Diet and Activity Promotion Trial (ADAPT) reported a 33% weight regain within a year of the end of the intervention [24] On the other hand, both the Diabetes Prevention Program (DPP) [25] and the Look AHEAD Trial showed maintenance of weight loss of 5%–7% over a 4 year follow-up period [26]. Follow-up meetings, education, and individualized plans are essential to improving body weight maintenance.
- *Exercise interventions in OA*: Historically, suggesting that a patient with OA should exercise might have seemed unwise or impossible due to increased joint pain and the notion that excessive movement might cause further joint damage.

    As a result of this, patients with OA would typically lead a sedentary lifestyle [21]. This has a detrimental impact on multiple aspects of their lives including both aerobic capacity and muscular strength. In the last few decades, exercise has become a valuable tool in the prevention and treatment of OA and is regularly included in treatment guidelines. Physical activity, of course, is an effective component of reducing body weight. In fact, weight loss of ≥3% is commonly observed, specifically when combined with diet [21,27]. (See also Chapter 5.)

    The Physical Activity Guidelines for Americans 2018 (PAGA 2018) Scientific Report recommended 150 minutes of moderate intensity physical activity as a way of both preventing and treating osteoarthritis [28]. Walking, which is the most common and readily available form of aerobic exercise, decreases pain from OA 26% and improved physical function (31%) within the short period of time of 8–12 weeks [29,30]. Long-term interventions are necessary in order to maintain these improvements.

16.3 RHEUMATOID ARTHRITIS

Rheumatoid arthritis (RA) is a chronic, progressive, autoimmune, inflammatory condition that affects the synovial joints [31]. Common symptoms include joint pain, swelling, and stiffness [32]. RA is associated with reduced life expectancy compared to the general population [33], largely due to increased prevalence and worse outcomes from cardiovascular disease (CVD) [34]. The cause for this remains unknown.

The chronic inflammation associated with RA can lead to the degradation of lean tissue, particularly muscle mass. In combination with an inactive lifestyle, this reduction in muscle mass frequently leads to increased accumulation of body fat and stable or slightly increased body weight. The etiology of RA is not clear. It is believed that RA is triggered when an immune genetically susceptible host is exposed to an antigen. This exposure triggers an initial inflammation which may initiate inflammation of the joints.

- *Obesity in RA*: It is not clear whether obesity predates or comes as a result of RA. However, the BMI reported in RA patients (ranging from 26.5 to 28.2 kg/m^2) is similar to that of the general population [35,36]. However, worldwide 18% of RA patients have obesity. In the United Kingdom, a higher prevalence of 31% of obesity in RA was found. Some early studies have suggested that obesity was found to associate with increased risk for developing RA. More recent studies, however, have not shown this association. Furthermore, whether or not obesity increases activity of RA is controversial. It should be noted that obesity, which is the well-established independent risk factor for CVD, also independently associates with other CVD risk factors in RA. In other words, RA patients with obesity are more likely to have CVD risk factors. Furthermore, it should be noted that the standard WHO criteria for overweight and obesity (i.e. overweight BMI 25–30 kg/m^2, obesity BMI > 30 kg/m^2) may not be technically correct for RA, given muscle wasting.
- *Causes of obesity and its control in RA*: Just as in the general population, energy intake and energy expenditure are the most significant predictors of obesity in RA [37]. These include low levels of physical activity and also inflammation. Increasing physical activity is therefore important for obesity control in RA patients as well as other populations. Whether or not there is any impact on standard dietary interventions for obesity is controversial in RA patients.

    With regard to exercise interventions, greater than 70% of RA patients do not perform any type of physical activity [38,39]. This may be the result of rheumatology health professionals adopting a traditional approach to recommend exercise restriction. However, it is now well established that well-designed physical exercise programs can promote prolonged improvements in RA without harmful effects on disease activity and joint damage. Increases in aerobic fitness and muscle mass in RA patients following well-designed training programs are comparable to those observed in the general population.

16.4 CONSIDERATIONS FOR WEIGHT LOSS INTERVENTIONS IN ARTHRITIC POPULATIONS

Both OA and RA patients can gain significant benefits from weight loss and optimum body composition. Of course, any interventions need to be planned with the specific needs of these patients in mind. Regular physical activity as part of an exercise program in patients with both OA and RA is essential to try to blunt any loss of lean muscle tissue. In RA patients, muscle wasting is prevalent and often clinically significant. Any caloric restriction needs to be closely monitored by individuals who are qualified in the treatment of RA.

16.5   CONSIDERATIONS FOR EXERCISE PRESCRIPTIONS IN ARTHRITIC POPULATIONS

Exercise prescription in populations with OA and RA is important but may be clinically challenging. It is clear that these patients respond to exercise in the same way and have the same potential for improvements in physical fitness and risk factor reduction as does the general population [40,41]. However, variation in the diseases such as different joints affected, flares, etc. should be taken into account when prescribing exercise for either OA or RA. This highlights the need for individualized exercise prescription. For example, patients may need a longer recovery period between exercise sessions if their disease is in the midst of a flare. Just as in other populations, patients should focus on exercising at a comfortable intensity and for a comfortable duration.

As with any weight loss or exercise, intervention adherence is very important. Behavioral strategies apply equally to patients with OA and RA as other patients. These considerations are outlined in more detail in Chapter 7.

16.6   SUMMARY/CONCLUSIONS

Arthritis is one of the leading causes of pain and disability worldwide. The most common form of arthritis is osteoarthritis (OA). This is strongly associated with obesity, particularly arthritis of the knee which may be a combination of mechanical forces, biomechanics, and inflammation. Rheumatoid arthritis (RA) has an immunologic component. Obesity is also associated with RA.

Weight loss in both OA and RA can contribute to a decrease in symptoms. However, most protocols should be geared to the specific clinical situation of each individual patient. In particular, exercise programs can lead to improvement in fitness and muscle strength. However, it is important, particularly in RA, that exercise prescription takes into account specific considerations related to the status of joints in RA patients.

CLINICAL APPLICATIONS

- Osteoarthritis of the knee is associated with obesity.
- Obesity may contribute to osteoarthritis both by mechanical considerations, biomechanics, and systemic inflammation.
- Obesity is also associated with rheumatoid arthritis.
- Regular exercise can benefit patients with both OA and RA. However, it should optimally be prescribed by clinicians who are familiar with the effects of exercise on the joints and must be individualized given the type of arthritis and associated symptoms in each patient.

REFERENCES

1. Stedman. *Stedman's Medical Dictionary.* 28th ed. Philadelphia, PA: Lippincott Williams and Wilkins; 2005.
2. Cotran R., Kumar V., Collins T. *Pathologic Basis of Disease.* 6th ed. Philadelphia, PA: W.B. Saunders Company; 1999.
3. Arthritis related statistics 2006. Accessed August 31, 2020. http://www.cdc.gov/arthritis/data_statistics/arthritis_related_stats.htm.
4. National Collaborating Centre for Chronic Conditions (UK): Osteoarthritis: National clinical guideline for care and management in adults. London: Royal College of Physicians (UK); 2008.
5. Nuki G. Osteoarthritis: A problem of joint failure. *Z Rheumatol* 1999, 58:142–147.
6. Valdes A., Spector T. The genetic epidemiology of osteoarthritis. *Curr Opin Rheumatol* 2010, 22:139–143.
7. Blagojevic M., Jinks C., Jeffery A., et al. Risk factors for onset of osteoarthritis of the knee in older adults: A systematic review and meta-analysis. *Osteoarthritis Cartilage* 2010; 18:24–33.
8. Stewart A., Black A: Bone mineral density in osteoarthritis. *Curr Opin Rheumatol* 2000; 12:464–467.
9. Bergink A., Uitterlinen A., Van Leeuwen J., et al. Bone mineral density and vertebral fracture history are associated with incident and progressive radiographic knee osteoarthritis in elderly men and women: The Rotterdam Study. *Bone.* 2005; 37:446–456.
10. Messier S. Obesity and osteoarthritis: Disease genesis and nonpharmacologic weight management. *Med Clin North Am.* 2009; 93:145–159.
11. Messier S. Obesity and osteoarthritis: Disease genesis and nonpharmacologic weight management. *Rheum Dis Clin North Am.* 2008; 34:713–729.
12. Leach R., Baumgard S., Broom J. Obesity: Its relationship to osteoarthritis of the knee. *Clin Orthop Relat Res.* 1973; 95:271–273.
13. Coggon D., Reading I., Croft P., et al. Knee osteoarthritis and obesity. *Int J Obes Relat Metab Disord.* 2001; 25:622–627.
14. Liu B., Balkwill A., Banks E., et al. Relationship of height, weight and body mass index to the risk of hip and knee replacements in middle-aged women. *Rheumatology (Oxford).* 2007; 46:861–867.
15. van Saase J., Vandenbroucke J., van Romunde L., et al. Osteoarthritis and obesity in the general population. A relationship calling for an explanation. *J Rheumatol.* 1988; 15:1152–1158.
16. Cooper C., Inskip H., Croft P., et al. Individual risk factors for hip osteoarthritis: Obesity, hip injury and physical activity. *Am J Epidemi.* 1998; 147:516–522.
17. Gravante G., Russo G., Pomara F., et al. Comparison of ground reaction forces between obese and control young adults during quiet standing on a baropodometric platform. *Clin Biomech.* 2003; 18:780–782.
18. Irving D., Cook J., Young M., et al. Obesity and pronated foot type may increase the risk of chronic plantar heel pain: A matched case-control study. *BMC Musculoskelet Disord.* 2007;8:41.
19. Riddle D., Pulisic M., Pidcoe P., et al. Risk factors for Plantar fasciitis: A matched case-control study. *J Bone Joint Surg Am.* 2003; 85:872–877.
20. Messier S., Ettinger W., Doyle T., et al. Obesity: Effects on gait in an osteoarthritic population. *J Appl Biomech.* 1996; 12:161–172.
21. Messier S. Diet and exercise for obese adults with knee osteoarthritis. *Clin Geriatr Med.* 2010; 26:461–477.
22. Felson D., Zhang Y., Anthony J., et al. Weight loss reduces the risk for symptomatic knee osteoarthritis in women. The Framingham Study. *Ann Intern Med.* 1992; 116:535–539.

23. Christensen R., Astrup A., Bliddal H. Weight loss: The treatment of choice for knee osteoarthritis? A randomized trial. *Osteoarthritis Cartilage.* 2005; 13:20–27.
24. Miller G., Rejeski W.J., Williamson J.D., et al. The arthritis, diet and activity promotion trial (ADAPT): Design, rationale, and baseline results. *Control Clin Trials.* 2003; 24(4):462–80.
25. The Diabetes Prevention Program Research Group. The Diabetes Prevention Program (DPP): Description of lifestyle intervention. *Diabetes Care.* 2002; 25:2165–2171.
26. Berger S., Huggins G., McCaffery J.M., et al. Comparison among criteria to define successful weight-loss maintainers and regainers in the action for health in diabetes (Look AHEAD) and Diabetes Prevention Program trials. *Am J Clinic Nutri.* 2017; 106:1337–1346.
27. Messier S., Loeser R., Mitchell M., et al. Exercise and weight loss in obese older adults with knee osteoarthritis: A preliminary study. *J Am Geriatr Soc.* 2000; 48:1062–1072.
28. 2018 Physical Activity Guidelines Advisory Committee. 2018 Physical Activity Guidelines Advisory Committee Scientific Report. Washington, DC: U.S. Department of Health and Human Services, 2018.
29. Minor M., Hewett J., Webel R., et al. Efficacy of physical conditioning exercise in patients with rheumatoid arthritis and osteoarthritis. *Arthritis Rheum.* 1989; 32:1396–1405.
30. Kovar P., Allegrante J., MacKenzie C., et al. Supervised fitness walking in patients with osteoarthritis of the knee. A randomized controlled trial. *Ann Intern Med.* 1992; 116:529–534.
31. Hunder G. *Atlas of Rheumatology.* 4th ed. Philadelphia, PA: Current Medicine; 2005.
32. Buch M., Emery P. The aetiology and pathogenesis of rheumatiod arthritis. *Hospital Pharmacist.* 2002; 9:5–10.
33. Erhardt C., Mumford P., Venables P., et al. Factors predicting a poor life prognosis in rheumatoid arthritis: An eight year prospective study. *Ann Rheum Dis.* 1989; 48:7–13.
34. Kitas G., Erb N. Tackling ischaemic heart disease in rheumatoid arthritis. *Rheumatology (Oxford).* 2003; 42:607–613.
35. Stavropoulos-Kalinoglou A., Metsios G., Koutedakis Y., et al. Redefining overweight and obesity in rheumatoid arthritis patients. *Ann Rheum Dis* 2007; 66:1316–1321.
36. Gordon M., Thomson E., Madhok R., et al. Can intervention modify adverse lifestyle variables in a rheumatoid population? Results of a pilot study. *Ann Rheum Dis.* 2002; 61:66–69.
37. Stavropoulos-Kalinoglou A., Metsios G., Smith J.P., et al. What predicts obesity in patients with rheumatoid arthritis? An investigation of the interactions between lifestyle and inflammation. *Int J Obes.* 2010; 34(2):295–301.
38. Ekdahl C., Broman G. Muscle strength, endurance, and aerobic capacity in rheumatoid arthritis: a comparative study with healthy subjects. *Ann Rheum Dis.* 1992; 51:35–40.
39. Scott D., Wolman R. Rest or exercise in inflammatory arthritis? *Br J Hosp Med.* 1992; 48:445–447.
40. Hakkinen A., Pakarinen A., Hannonen P., et al. Effects of prolonged combined strength and endurance training on physical fitness, body composition and serum hormones in women with rheumatoid arthritis and in healthy controls. *Clin Exp Rheumatol.* 2005; 23:505–512.
41. Cooney J., Law R., Matschke V., et al. Benefits of exercise in rheumatoid arthritis. *J Aging Res.* 2011; 2011: 681640.

Section III

---

*Future Directions and
Public Health Issues*

17 Beyond Subcutaneous Fat

James M. Rippe, MD
Rippe Lifestyle Institute
University of Massachusetts Medical School

CONTENTS

17.1 INTRODUCTION

The obesity pandemic is a public health concern for countries around the world. As a result of this, considerable research has taken place exploring the health consequences of adipose tissue. A key finding has been that adipose tissue functions like an endocrine organ. Furthermore, the importance of the distribution of body fat has been documented and methods for assessing it have been developed and are increasingly being utilized.

Obesity is a major risk factor for cardiovascular disease (CVD), type 2 diabetes mellitus (T2DM), metabolic syndrome (MetS), and insulin resistance. However, it should be pointed out that not every patient with obesity has insulin resistance or is at high risk for T2DM and CVD [1]. It has been recognized over several decades that metabolic abnormalities which underlie the MetS are more strongly associated with central fat rather than total adiposity. Furthermore, intraabdominal adipose tissue (IAAT) and liver fat are key determinants of metabolic abnormalities [2].

More important than how much fat a person stores is where he/she stores it as well as whether the volume of excess energy to be stored exceeds the capacity of the adipocytes to store it. Indeed, abdominal obesity is increasingly understood to play a major role in a variety of pathophysiologic conditions associated with central

DOI: 10.1201/9781003099116-20

adiposity [3–7]. These include the risks for coronary heart disease (CHD), T2DM, hypertension, and atherosclerosis.

Many researchers now feel that visceral adiposity may be more important than the diagnosis of obesity using body mass index (BMI). Viseral abdominal obesity as a core component of MetS is now recognized by a variety of medical organizations and is incorporated into most definitions of MetS. For example, it is incorporated into the most widely MetS diagnostic criteria developed by the National Cholesterol Education Program-ATP III (NCEP-ATP III) [8]. Ectopic fat, which is fat stored outside of normal deposition within adipocyte cells, can occur in places like the liver or within muscles and further exacerbates its risks. Even within the normal range of BMI, the accumulation of visceral fat constitutes an independent cardiovascular risk. It is clear that body shape and location of adipose tissue have enormous cardiometabolic implications.

17.2   CENTRAL ABDOMINAL OBESITY

Waist circumference and BMI are normally correlated on a population level. However, there is substantial individual variation in waist circumference from one patient to another with similar BMI values [2]. Since in some instances BMI correlates more strongly with health risk than does waist circumference and vice versa, it is important that clinicians measure both BMI and waist circumference. (See also Chapters 2 and 4.)

Accumulated fat in the intraabdominal or visceral depots is strongly associated with obesity-related complications. Waist circumference correlates with visceral fat as measured by abdominal CT scanning and also with risk factors for coronary heart disease such as hypertension and dyslipidemia as well as hyperglycemia. For this reason, the NCEP-ATP III lists increased waist circumference as a major component of the diagnostic criteria for MetS [8]. This is marked by waist circumference exceeding 40 inches (102 cm) in men and greater than 35 inches (88 cm) in women. (See also Chapter 14.)

- *Relationship between central obesity and cardiovascular disease*: Multiple studies have shown that increased waist circumference or waist-to-hip ratio (WHR) strongly predict CHD. Some studies have shown that all-cause mortality is also increased by 3% over 4.5 years for every increased centimeter of waist circumference in patients with coronary artery disease [9]. It should be noted that even though a combination of waist circumference and BMI more accurately predict CVD risk and risk of T2DM than BMI alone, there still is considerable variation between IAAT and intrahepatic lipid (IHCL) depots.

17.3   VISCERAL ADIPOSITY

Fat accumulation around and inside intraabdominal solid organs is referred to as visceral or intraabdominal fat. Portions of the visceral fat – mesenteric and omental adipose depot – are drained by the hepatic portal vein which delivers nutrient-rich blood to the liver. Retroperitoneal and subcutaneous abdominal depots are non-portal depots.

- *Visceral fat*: Accumulation of intraabdominal fat increases hepatic adipose tissue, insulin resistance (IR), and metabolic abnormalities such as glucose intolerance, low HDL cholesterol, elevated triglycerides (TGs), and hypertension. IR is the fundamental etiology [10–12]. A number of studies have shown a strong relationship between intraabdominal fat accumulation and IR. In addition to adipocytes found in abdominal adipose tissue, there are also macrophages which produce pro-inflammatory cytokines such a tumor necrosis factor alpha (TNFα) and IL-6 [13]. IR is thought to underlie diabetes and contribute to the ectopic storage of lipids in the liver, skeletal muscle, and pancreatic island cells.
- *Lipid metabolism and visceral adiposity*: Visceral adiposity is associated with serum levels of small dense LDL cholesterol and high Apo-B [14], hypertriglyceridemia, and reduced HDL cholesterol [15]. In dyslipidemic patients, intraabdominal fat volume correlates with hepatic cholesterol synthesis.
- *Sex and continent of origin effects*: There are ethnic and sex differences in the rate of accumulation of visceral fat and its relevance to metabolic disease. In particular, men of East Asian or European ancestry seem particularly prone to accumulating visceral fat [16]. Furthermore, men have greater IAAT than women [17,18]. However, this difference is weakest in African Americans. Many factors contribute to determine the volume of visceral fat including the balance of sex hormones such as free testosterone, growth hormone, IGF-1, as well as dietary intake of sucrose and saturated fat, and lack of physical activity [19]. Age is also a significant factor with older individuals having larger amounts of visceral fat than younger individuals [20].
- *Genetic factors*: There appears to be considerable variation in gene expression and secretory products in visceral fat [21]. A wide variety of genetic research projects are ongoing in this area, although this area of research is in its infancy.
- *Assessment of intraabdominal adipose tissue*: Adipose tissue contains adipocytes, macrophages, connective tissue, and blood vessels and is not identical to adipose fat which refers only to stored TGs. Body fat has traditionally been divided into subcutaneous, intramuscular, and visceral fat [22]. The gold standard for measuring visceral fat has been abdominal computed tomography (CT) (at the L4-L5 level) as well as magnetic resonance imaging (MRI). Unfortunately, CT and MRI are not widely used clinically because of the limitations of cost and radiation exposure.
- *Anthropomorphic measurement*: Waist circumference and WHR are typically used in epidemiologic studies to indirectly estimate intraabdominal fat volume. Even though these measures correlate with IAAT, when measured by CT scanning they are less accurate. Waist circumference is actually a better reflection of intraabdominal fat volume than WHR [23,24]. Furthermore, waist circumference is the easiest anthropomorphic measurement for health

care professionals to use to diagnose abdominal adiposity and get at least an estimate of visceral fat volume.

- *Dual-energy X-ray absorptiometry*: Dual-energy X-ray absorptiometry (DEXA) was initially utilized to examine bone mineral density but can also accurately measure total body fat and regional fat distribution [24]. DEXA is more accurate than anthropomorphic measured and more practical and cost effective than CT or MRI scans. A shortcoming of DEXA is that it cannot distinguish between subcutaneous and visceral abdominal fat deposits.

- *Abdominal ultrasonography*: Abdominal ultrasonography imaging may also be suitable for intraabdominal fat measurements. Some technical issues such as establishing a universally followed protocol for positioning the ultrasound probe and for timing the measurement with regard to the respiratory cycle potentially hampers this technique [23]. It is recommended that ultrasound measurements be performed at the end for quiet inspiration and by compressing the transducer against the abdomen, given the distortion of the abdominal cavity during scanning.

17.4   PERIPHERAL FAT DOES NO HARM

Peripheral fat mass (PFM) which is fat deposited subcutaneously below the waist and around the arms has no defined physiologic roles beyond the traditional one of energy storage. In a variety of studies, PFM actually showed an independent negative correlation with glucose, atherogenic lipid, and MetS as well arterial stiffness and aortic calcification [25,26]. In women, fat accumulation in the gluteal and femoral regions actually may possess some degree of protection from CVD. It has been argued that adequate PFM reduces the need for fat storage in central, intraabdominal, and ectopic deposits. Surgical removal of large amounts of subcutaneous fat by liposuction in a group of diabetic and nondiabetic individuals did not improve insulin sensitivity in muscle, liver, or adipose tissue and did not change plasma concentrations of circulating mediators of inflammation.

- *Biological differences – visceral versus subcutaneous body fat*: A number of biological differences occur between visceral and subcutaneous body fat [27]. From an anatomical point of view, visceral fat is present mainly in the mesentery and omentum and drains directly through the portal circulation to the liver. Visceral fat is also more cellular, vascular, and innervate; contains a large number of inflammatory and immune cells; and contains a larger percent of large adipocytes when compared to subcutaneous adipose tissue [28]. The propensity for adipocyte hypertrophy differs by depot. In obese women, hyperplasia is predominant in the subcutaneous fat depot. Whereas fat cell hypertrophy is observed in both the omentum and subcutaneous compartments. In men, omental adipocyte size plateaus in the upper two tertiles of waist circumference (waist circumference above 125 cm). Men have larger adipocytes in all intraabdominal depots compared to women.

    It should be noted that some individuals display "benign" obesity characterized by normal insulin sensitivity and low levels of ectopic fat (liver and muscle) as compared to peers with equal amounts of obesity [29]. This would appear to be a result of different concentrations of inflammatory and other markers released by IAAT. The mechanism of differences between individuals with "benign" obesity and peers with equal amounts of obesity who have more metabolic abnormalities is not completely known.

17.5 NON-ALCOHOLIC FATTY LIVER DISEASE

The prevalence of non-alcoholic fatty liver disease (NAFLD) has risen dramatically in the past 20 years, similar to the rise in obesity [30]. NAFLD is now the leading cause of liver failure and liver transplantations in the world. In NAFLD, liver biopsy reveals steatosis (fatty droplets) and inflammation of the liver lobes. Non-alcoholic steatosis (NASH) is part of a spectrum of NAFLD which includes simple fatty liver (fat droplets causing the ballooning of hepatocytes and inflammation) and NAFLD-associated fibrosis (extracellular deposition of type 1 and type 3 collagen) and cirrhosis (replacement of liver tissue by fibrosis scar tissue and nodules) [31].

Greater than 5% of liver volume as fat defines steatosis and 30% of fat is the cutoff for liver transplantation donors [31]. Historically, NAFLD has affected 2%–24% of the general population and with men more prevalent than women typically found after the age of 30 [32]. It should be noted, however, that NAFLD can be found in youth with obesity. In morbid obesity patients (BMI greater than 35 kg/m^2), up to 90% have NAFLD with advanced disease in 9%–40% [33,34]. The severity of NAFLD cannot be predicted by subcutaneous adiposity distribution.

- *Fatty liver*: The presence of fatty liver in persons with BMI greater than 30 is estimated to be twice that of the general population [35]. Visceral adiposity is highly correlated with hepatic fat, and hepatic fat content has been found to be responsible for elevated CVD risk. Leptin, adiponectin, and TNFα may play a role in the progression of fatty liver disease. NAFLD is also clearly associated with T2DM [36]. In addition, NASH may play a role in carcinogenesis. NASH patients have approximately ten times higher rate of hepatocellular carcinoma compared to the general U.S. population.
- *Development of non-alcoholic liver disease*: How NAFLD develops is not well understood. It has been postulated that the dysregulation of fatty acid metabolism (resulting in lipotoxicity) is followed by hepatocyte necrosis [37]. This, in turn, is followed by oxidative stress and increase in inflammatory mediators. Inflammation is considered to be a driving force behind NASH. Indeed, visceral adipose tissue creates a state of low-grade inflammation in 75% of patients [38]. Blood triglyceride (TG) levels of greater than 150 mg/dl are often present in NASH, and decreases in adiponectin are also strongly correlated with NASH.
- *Portal vein connection*: The hepatic portal vein collects venous blood from the stomach, small intestines, pancreas, and spleen and drains the omental and mesenteric adipose tissue depots associated with these organs [39]. Thus, the inclination of IAAT to store TGs and release fatty acids directly affects the liver. Also, other adipokines and other factors are expressed at a higher level than in IAAT.

- *Imaging the liver*: Simple steatosis is detected by imaging studies (e.g. CT, MRI, or MRS), while the confirmation of NASH in this staging requires a liver biopsy. Since liver biopsy is invasive, techniques such as ultrasound, CT, magnetic resonance spectroscopy (MRS), and MRI-based protocols have been developed. MRS is the preferred imaging method [40].

17.6   ARE WEIGHT GAIN, ABDOMINAL OBESITY, AND DEVELOPMENT OF FATTY LIVER A ONE-WAY STREET?

Early-stage fatty liver, which is the most common form of NAFLD, is reversible. In addition, strategies that enable and maintain weight loss have also been shown to yield positive results. Some studies have shown that short-term weight reduction programs will yield moderate reduction in visceral fat and create benefits in lipid profile, insulin sensitivity, and blood pressure, similar to that observed after a major weight reduction [41]. Of note, most of the fat loss in the first 2 weeks of caloric restriction and exercise is from visceral fat.

- *Diet*: The Look AHEAD Trial (Action for Health and Diabetes) studied over 5,000 individuals with obesity or who are overweight with type 2 diabetes. Average weight loss across 4 years in the intensive lifestyle intervention arm (−6.2%) exceeded that observed in the control arm of diabetes support and education [42]. A sub-study showed that there were substantial reductions in abdominal fat cells and an increase in insulin sensitivity [43]. In another sub-study after 12 months, only 3% of lifestyle intervention subjects compared to 26% of control group developed steatosis [44]. Other studies have confirmed similar findings.
- *Exercise*: Individuals who are physically active develop smaller IAAT. In one study, a model of regular physical exercise (30 minutes of vigorous exercise two to four times a week) resulted in a 7.4% reduction in IAAT [45]. It has been argued that increase in IAAT with aging is due at least in part to a steady decline in high intensity (vigorous) exercise as individuals age.
- *Drugs*: Thiazolidinediones (TZDs) that are used to treat IR and T2DMs also can reduce visceral adiposity. Combinations of medicines that enhance satiety and reduce food intake (e.g. Glucagon-like peptide-1 analogues) together with exercise and caloric reduction can also reduce NASH [46].
- *Bariatric surgery*: Dietary restriction prior to surgery can shrink the size of the liver and make surgery technically easier. The most commonly performed bariatric surgery procedures (gastric banding and gastric bypass) decrease body weight and reverse T2DM in 62%–83% of patients. However, there are no data regarding NAFLD effects [47].
- *Therapies for NASH*: There are no treatments for NASH approved by the American Association for the Study of Liver Disease [48]. However, their anecdotal reports suggest that both diet and physical activity can reverse simple steatosis. In one cross-sectional study, survey of 812 patients with NAFLD vigorous exercise decreased the risk of finding NASH by 35%.

17.7   OTHER ECTOPIC DEPOTS

It has been hypothesized that insufficient adipocytes or limited capacity promote ectopic depot of fat [49]. This is an area of active research.

17.8   SUMMARY/CONCLUSIONS

It is clear that visceral fat is different from peripheral fat in terms of its metabolic effects. Visceral adiposity can lead to a variety of metabolic derangements including insulin resistance, fatty liver, and, ultimately, non-alcoholic fatty liver disease. For this reason, it is important for clinicians to focus not only on overall obesity but also on the location of added fat. A variety of tools are available to assist in this process.

PRACTICAL APPLICATIONS

- Both degree of adiposity and location of fat are important to assess the risk of cardiovascular disease and type 2 diabetes.
- Both BMI and waist circumference should, therefore, be measured in all patients with obesity.
- Patients with obesity who have metabolic abnormalities obtaining additional tests to assess liver fat (e.g. DEXA) may be very useful and should be considered by clinicians treating patients with obesity.

REFERENCES

1. Despres J., Lemieux I. Abdominal obesity and metabolic syndrome. *Nature.* 2006;444/7121: 881–887.
2. Despres J. Excess visceral adipose tissue/ectopic fat the missing link in the obesity paradox? *J Am Coll Cardiol.* 2011;57/19: 1887–1889.
3. Zamboni M., Armellini F., Sheiban I., et al. Relation of body fat distribution in men and degree of coronary narrowings in coronary artery disease. *Am J Cardiol.* 1992;70/13: 1135–1138.
4. Bjorntorp P. Abdominal obesity and the development of noninsulin-dependent diabetes mellitus. *Diabetes Metab Rev.* 1988;4/6: 615–622.
5. Folsom A., Kaye S., Sellers T., et al. Body fat distribution and 5-year risk of death in older women. *JAMA.* 1993;269/4: 483–487.
6. Folsom A., Prineas R., Kaye S., et al. Incidence of hypertension and stroke in relation to body fat distribution and other risk factors in older women. *Stroke.* 1990;21/5: 701–706.
7. Price G., Uauy R., Breeze E., et al. Weight, shape, and mortality risk in older persons: Elevated waist-hip ratio, not high body mass index, is associated with a greater risk of death. *Am J Clin Nutr.* 2006;84/2: 449–460.
8. Grundy S., Cleeman J., Daniels S., et al. Diagnosis and management of the metabolic syndrome: an American Heart Association/National Heart, Lung, and Blood Institute Scientific Statement. *CIRC.* 2005;112/17: 2735–2752.
9. Kanhai D., Kappelle L., van der Graaf Y., et al. The risk of general and abdominal adiposity in the occurrence of new vascular events and mortality in patients with various manifestations of vascular disease. *Int J Obes. (Lond).* 2011;36:695.
10. Walton C., Lees B., Crook D., Godsland I.F., Stevenson J.C. Relationships between insulin metabolism, serum lipid profile, body fat distribution and blood pressure in healthy men. *Atherosclerosis.* 1995;118/1: 35–43.

11. Kahn B., Flier J. Obesity and insulin resistance. *J Clin Invest.* 2000;106/4: 473–481.
12. Miyazaki Y., DeFronzo R. Visceral fat dominant distribution in male type 2 diabetic patients is closely related to hepatic insulin resistance, irrespective of body type. *Cardiovasc Diabetol.* 2009;8: 44.
13. Bremer A.A., Devaraj S., Afify A., Jialal I. Adipose tissue dysregulation in patients with metabolic syndrome. *J Clin Endocrinol Metab.* 2011;96: E1782.
14. Despres J., Moorjani S., Lupien P., et al. Regional distribution of body fat, plasma lipoproteins, and cardiovascular disease. *Arterio.* 1990;10/4: 497–511.
15. Lupattelli G., Pirro M., Mannarino M., et al. Visceral fat positively correlates with cholesterol synthesis in dyslipidaemic patients. *Eur J Clin Invest.* 2011;42: 164.
16. Hill J., Sidney S., Lewis C., et al. Racial differences in amounts of visceral adipose tissue in young adults: the CARDIA (Coronary Artery Risk Development in Young Adults) study. *Am J Clin Nutr.* 1999;69/3: 381–387.
17. Demerath E , Sun S., Rogers N., et al. Anatomical patterning of visceral adipose tissue: Race, sex, and age variation. *Obesity (Silver Spring).* 2007;15/12: 2984–2993.
18. Liu J., Fox C., Hickson D., et al. Impact of abdominal visceral and subcutaneous adipose tissue on cardiometabolic risk factors: The Jackson heart study. *J Clin Endocrinol Metab.* 2010;95/12: 5419–5426.
19. Hamdy O., Porramatikul S., Al-Ozairi E. Metabolic obesity: The paradox between visceral and subcutaneous fat. *Curr Diabetes Rev.* 2006;2/4: 367–373.
20. Kuk J., Saunders T., Davidson L., et al. Age-related changes in total and regional fat distribution. *Ageing Res Rev.* 2009;8/4: 339–348.
21. Perusse L., Rice T., Chagnon Y., et al. A genome-wide scan for abdominal fat assessed by computed tomography in the Quebec Family Study. *Diabetes.* 2001;50/3: 614–621.
22. Chowdhury B., Sjostrom L., Alpsten M., et al. A multicompartment body composition technique based on computerized tomography. *Int J Obes Relat Metab Disord.* 1994;18/4: 219–234.
23. van der Kooy K., Seidell J. Techniques for the measurement of visceral fat: A practical guide. *Int J Obes Relat Metab Disord.* 1993;17/4: 187–196.
24. Van Pelt R., Evans E., Schechtman K., et al. Contributions of total and regional fat mass to risk for cardiovascular disease in older women. *Am J Physiol Endocrinol Metab.* 2002;282/5: E1023–E1028.
25. Lissner L., Bjorkelund C., Heitmann B., et al. Larger hip circumference independently predicts health and longevity in a Swedish female cohort. *Obes Res.* 2001;9/10: 644–646.
26. Faloia E., Tirabassi G., Canibus P., et al. Protective effect of leg fat against cardiovascular risk factors in obese premenopausal women. *Nutr Metab Cardiovasc Dis.* 2009;19/1: 39–44.
27. Ibrahim M. Subcutaneous and visceral adipose tissue: Structural and functional differences. *Obes Rev.* 2010;11/1: 11–18.
28. Ohman M., Wright A., Wickenheiser K., et al. Visceral adipose tissue and atherosclerosis. *Curr Vasc Pharmacol.* 2009;7/2: 169–179.
29. Stefan N., Kantartzis K., Machann J., et al. Identification and characterization of metabolically benign obesity in humans. *Arch Intern Med.* 2008;168/15: 1609–1616.
30. Ludwig J., Viggiano T., McGill D., et al. Nonalcoholic steatohepatitis: Mayo Clinic experiences with a hitherto unnamed disease. *Mayo Clin Proc.* 1980;55/7: 434–438.
31. Busuttil R., Tanaka K. The utility of marginal donors in liver transplantation. *Liver Transpl.* 2003;9/7: 651–663.
32. Sagi R., Reif S., Neuman G., et al. Nonalcoholic fatty liver disease in overweight children and adolescents. *Acta Paediatr.* 2007;96/8: 1209–1213.
33. Scheen A.J., Luyckx F.H., Desaive C., Lefebvre P.J. Severe/extreme obesity: A medical disease requiring a surgical treatment? *Acta Clin Belg.* 1999;54/3: 154–161.

34. Gholam P.M., Flancbaum L., Machan J.T., Charney D.A., Kotler D.P. Nonalcoholic fatty liver disease in severely obese subjects. *Am J Gastroenterol.* 2007;102/2: 399–408.
35. Buechler C., Wanninger J., Neumeier M. Adiponectin, a key adipokine in obesity related liver diseases. *World J Gastroenterol.* 2011;17/23: 2801–2811.
36. Kashyap S., Diab D., Baker A., et al. Triglyceride levels and not adipokine concentrations are closely related to severity of nonalcoholic fatty liver disease in an obesity surgery cohort. *Obesity (Silver Spring).* 2009;17/9: 1696–1701.
37. Day C., James O. Steatohepatitis: A tale of two "hits"? *Gastroenterology.* 1998;114/4: 842–845.
38. Farb M., Bigornia S., Mott M., et al. Reduced adipose tissue inflammation represents an intermediate cardiometabolic phenotype in obesity. *J Am Coll Cardiol.* 2011;58/3: 232–237.
39. Shah V., Kamath P. Portal hypertension and gastrointestinal bleeding. In: Feldman M., Friedman L.S., Brandt L.J. (eds.) *Sleisenger and Fordtran's Gastrointestinal and Liver Disease: Pathophysiology, Diagnosis, Management.* Saunders Elsevier, Philadelphia, PA, 2010.
40. Reeder S., Sirlin C. Quantification of liver fat with magnetic resonance imaging. *Magn Reson Imaging Clin N Am.* 2010;18/3: 337–57.
41. Brochu M., Tchernof A., Turner A., et al. Is there a threshold of visceral fat loss that improves the metabolic profile in obese postmenopausal women? *Metabolism.* 2003;52/5: 599–604.
42. Wing R. Long-term effects of a lifestyle intervention on weight and cardiovascular risk factors in individuals with type 2 diabetes mellitus: four-year results of the Look AHEAD trial. *Arch Intern Med.* 2010;170/17: 1566–1575.
43. Pasarica M., Tchoukalova Y., Heilbronn L., et al. Differential effect of weight loss on adipocyte size subfractions in patients with type 2 diabetes. *Obesity (Silver Spring).* 2009;17/10: 1976–1978.
44. Lazo M., Solga S., Horska A., et al. Effect of a 12-month intensive lifestyle intervention on hepatic steatosis in adults with type 2 diabetes. *Diab Care.* 2010;33/10: 2156–2163.
45. Hairston K., Vitolins M., Norris J., et al. Lifestyle factors and 5-year abdominal fat accumulation in a minority cohort: The IRAS family study. *Obesity (Silver Spring).* 2011;20: 421.
46. Mitri J., Hamdy O. Diabetes medications and body weight. *Expert Opin Drug Saf.* 2009;8/5: 573–584.
47. O'Brien P. Bariatric surgery: Mechanisms, indications and outcomes. *J Gastroenterol Hepatol.* 2010;25/8: 1358–1365.
48. Sanyal A., Brunt E., Kleiner D., et al. Endpoints and clinical trial design for nonalcoholic steatohepatitis. *Hepatology.* 2011;54/1: 344–353.
49. Heilbronn L., Smith S., Ravussin E. Failure of fat cell proliferation, mitochondrial function and fat oxidation results in ectopic fat storage, insulin resistance and type II diabetes mellitus. *Int J Obes Relat Metab Disord.* 2004;28/Suppl 4: S12–S21.

18 Public Health and Obesity

James M. Rippe, MD
Rippe Lifestyle Institute
University of Massachusetts Medical School

CONTENTS

18.1 INTRODUCTION

Given the high level of prevalence of obesity both in the United States and the rest of the world and its association with multiple other significant metabolic abnormalities, it is important to find ways of addressing this epidemic. Since individual approaches have largely not been successful, communities have sought to implement more broad-based policy and environmental efforts to address behaviors and environment that contribute to obesity. These include initiatives in healthy eating, active living, and decreased sedentary behavior.

Some successes have been achieved both by states and local communities in developing a number of supports in the environment and also in public policy to encourage healthy eating and active living.

An increasing amount of evidence now exists to guide public health and community leaders in efforts to seek the most efficacious plans to prevent obesity [1,2]. Nonetheless, more efforts are still needed to evaluate specific policy and interventional changes and their impact on weight gain and obesity. The Centers for Disease Control and Prevention (CDC) has published a set of "common community measures for obesity prevention" [3]. This report seeks to bring together in one place, identify and recommend a set of obesity prevention strategies, and recommend measurements

DOI: 10.1201/9781003099116-21

that local governments and communities can use to plan, implement, and monitor initiatives to prevent obesity. These guidelines are found in Table 18.1.

Public policy and environmental supports in developing and initiating effective public health programming have been shown to be successful in a number of public health challenges. These same tools are now being applied in the area of obesity prevention. The current chapter will focus on how various health policies and policy informed environmental supports at both national, state, and local have been applied to help address the ongoing worldwide pandemic of obesity.

18.2   AGRICULTURE AND FOOD SUPPLY POLICIES THAT SUPPORT HEALTHY EATING

Healthy eating is essential for overall good health and vital to reducing the prevalence of overweight and obesity. Following a diet with adequate fruits and vegetables along with other nutritious foods can help reduce the risk of many of the leading causes of illness and death including obesity, diabetes, some cancers, CVD, and T2DM.

Unfortunately, few adults in the United States meet the recommendations of the US Department of Health and Human Services and the US Department of Agriculture (USDA 2020 Dietary Guidelines for Americans). Less than 10% of adults meet the intake recommendations for vegetables, and 12% of adults meet the recommendations for fruit [4].

Many environmental factors impact healthy eating. Penchansky and Thomas developed a conceptual model that includes dimensions relevant to healthy eating [5]. These include availability, affordability, acceptability, and accommodation.

Availability includes concepts such as whether nutritious foods are available to individuals and families. Food deserts are common in the United States. These are areas where adequate access to fruits and vegetables, whole grains, and low-fat dairy products are not readily available [6,7]. The USDA defines a food desert as one which includes the key components of low access such as community, number of individuals impacted, and distance an individual lives from a supermarket or grocery store.

It is important that clinicians understand and are aware of the fact that preventive recommendations may be difficult to follow for individuals who have little access to nutritious or affordable foods. In addition, oftentimes, nutritious and healthy diets are more expensive than processed foods which creates an extra impediment to following nutritional guidelines [8].

There is also an issue of whether or not nutritious foods meet cultural norms and are acceptable to individuals. The issue of accommodation relates to the number of hours that stores are open.

The issue of accessibility also involves distance to a food store in relation to components of the diet such as fruits and vegetable consumption. Access to an automobile also plays a significant role in accessibility.

Efforts have been made in various Farm Bills to try to positively affect the food supply in the United States. Over 50% of funds approved in Farm Bills are typically allocated to nutrition/healthy eating programs. This includes national school lunch programs, community food security, promotional farmers' markets, fruit and vegetable consumption, and the Supplemental Nutrition Action Program (SNAP) [9]. In

TABLE 18.1

Summary of Recommended Community Policy Strategies and Measurements to Prevent Obesity

Strategies to Promote the Availability of Affordable Healthy Food and Beverages

Strategy	Communities should increase the availability of healthier food and beverage choices in public service venues.
Suggested measurement	A policy exists to apply nutrition standards that are consistent with the dietary guidelines for Americans (US Department of Health and Human Services, US Department of Agriculture. Dietary guidelines for Americans. 6th ed. Washington, DC: U.S. Government Printing Office; 2005.) to all food sold (e.g. meal menus and vending machines) within local government facilities in a local jurisdiction or on public school campuses during the school day within the largest school district in a local jurisdiction.
Strategy	Communities should improve the availability of affordable healthier food and beverage choices in public service venues.
Suggested measurement	A policy exists to affect the cost of healthier foods and beverages (as defined by the Institute of Medicine [IOM] [Institute of Medicine. *Preventing childhood obesity: health in the balance.* Washington, DC: The National Academies Press; 2005]) relative to the cost of less healthy foods and beverages sold within local government facilities in a local jurisdiction or on public school campuses during the school day within the largest school district in a local jurisdiction.
Strategy	Communities should provide incentives for the production, distribution, and procurement of foods from local farms.
Suggested measurement	Local government has a policy that encourages the production, distribution, or procurement of food from local farms in the local jurisdiction.

Strategies to Support Healthy Food and Beverage Choices

Strategy	Communities should restrict the availability of less healthy foods and beverages in public service venues.
Suggested measurement	A policy exists that prohibits the sale of less healthy foods and beverages (as defined by IOM [Institute of Medicine. *Preventing childhood obesity: health in the balance.* Washington, DC: The National Academies Press; 2005]) within local government facilities in a local jurisdiction or on public school campuses during the school day within the largest school district in a local jurisdiction.
Strategy	Communities should institute smaller portion size options in public service venues.
Suggested measurement	Local government has a policy to limit the portion size of any entree (including sandwiches and entrée salads) by either reducing the standard portion size of entrees or offering smaller portion sizes in addition to standard portion sizes within local government facilities within a local jurisdiction.
Strategy	Communities should limit advertisements of less healthy foods and beverages.

(*Continued*)

TABLE 18.1 *(Continued)*
Summary of Recommended Community Policy Strategies and Measurements to Prevent Obesity

Suggested measurement	A policy exists that limits advertising and promotion of less healthy foods and beverages within local government facilities in a local jurisdiction or on public school campuses during the school day within the largest school district in a local jurisdiction.
Strategy	Communities should discourage the consumption of sugar-sweetened beverages.
Suggested measurement	Licensed child care facilities within the local jurisdiction are required to ban sugar-sweetened beverages, including flavored/sweetened milk, and limit the portion size of 100% juice.

Strategy to Encourage Breastfeeding

Strategy	Communities should increase support for breastfeeding.
Suggested measurement	Local government has a policy requiring local government facilities to provide breastfeeding accommodations for employees that include both time and private space for breastfeeding during working hours.

Strategies to Encourage Physical Activity or Limit Sedentary Activity Among Children and Youth

Strategy	Communities should require physical education in schools.
Suggested measurement	The largest school district located within the local jurisdiction has a policy that requires a minimum of 150 minutes per week of PE in public elementary schools and a minimum of 225 minutes per week of PE in public middle schools and high schools throughout the school year (as recommended by the National Association of Sports and Physical Education).
Strategy	Communities should increase the amount of physical activity in PE programs in schools.
Suggested measurement	The largest school district located within the local jurisdiction has a policy that requires K-12 students to be physically active for at least 50% of time spent in PE classes in public schools.

Strategies to Create Safe Communities That Support Physical Activity

Strategy	Communities should support locating schools within easy walking distance of residential areas.
Suggested measurement	The largest school district in the local jurisdiction has a policy that supports locating new schools, and/or repairing or expanding existing schools, within easy walking or biking distance of residential areas.
Strategy	Communities should enhance traffic safety in areas where persons are or could be physically active.
Suggested Measurement	Local government has a policy for designing and operating streets with safe access for all users which includes at least one element suggested by the national complete streets coalition (http://www.completestreets.org).

Adapted from: Centers for Disease Control. MMWR 58(RRr-7) 2009. https://www.cdc.gov/mmwr/pdf/rr/rr5807.pdf.

addition, Farm Bills typically allocate 15% of funds to subsidize soybean and corn products. These crops are less expensive and used more often in food production, thereby lowering costs of many foods.

In 2008, the Farm Bill provided 1.3 billion dollars in new funding over 10 years for growing fruits, vegetables, and nuts. On the state level, the 2008 Farm Bill provided 500 million dollars towards the provision of fresh fruit and/or vegetables and snacks in schools and allowed schools to have a greater variety and choice of buying food from local farmers. The Nutrition Program for Women, Infants and Children (WIC) has developed a community-based effort where participants receive $10 vouchers for fresh produce. This has been demonstrated to increase consumption of fruits and vegetables compared to a control group. This effect lasted 6 months during the initial testing following the intervention.

All of these nutritional initiatives are important as supports for healthy eating which, in turn, plays a significant role in helping to lower the prevalence of weight gain and obesity.

18.3 SUPPORTS FOR A PHYSICALLY ACTIVE LIFESTYLE

Regular physical activity is one of the most powerful ways of lowering the risk of weight gain and obesity [10]. While physical activity by itself may not be a powerful mechanism for initial weight loss, it is absolutely essential for long-term maintenance of weight loss. Moreover, physical inactivity is a significant independent risk factor for chronic diseases including obesity, CVD, T2DM, and cancer. Interventions that increase physical activity are critical components in the prevention and management of chronic diseases. Policy and environmental approaches to promoting physical activity have been demonstrated to be effective and significant reinforcers for clinicians to counsel and advise all of their patients to be more physically active. This is particularly important for individuals who have gained weight or are obese.

A number of different settings have been employed in this area including school settings, worksites, community organizations, public recreational facilities, and parks. Environmental infrastructure – both the built environment and the natural environment – can also provide opportunities for people to participate in active transport, active sport, and recreation. All of these are important modalities for community involvement to lower the risk of weight gain and obesity on a population-wide level.

18.3.1 SCHOOL SETTINGS

Walking and bicycling to and from school have been demonstrated to increase physical activity among children as part of active transport [11]. The increase in energy expenditure during transport has the potential to improve energy balance and help ameliorate overweight and obesity. It should be noted, however, that the number of people walking or bicycling to and from school has dropped significantly over the past 40 years [12]. This is due, in part, to the increased distance between children's homes and school. It has been argued that as new schools are built, considering locating schools in areas close to residential areas represents a good strategy.

18.3.2   School-Based Food Policy

School-based food policies such as limiting soda, juice drinks, energy drinks, and sports drinks may also be an effective strategy to help children and adolescents from overconsuming calories. It has been demonstrated in several research trials that these strategies have resulted in decreased consumption of sugar-sweetened beverages [13]. In addition to the strategy of reducing access to sugary drinks, increasing access to fresh fruits and vegetables has also been demonstrated to be effective in increasing the consumption of such foods.

18.3.3   School-Based Physical Activity Policies

A significant number of states mandate some level of physical activity in schools: 36 states mandate physical education (PE) for elementary school students, 33 states mandate PE for middle school students, and 42 mandate PE for high school students [14]. The implementation of quality PE classes in schools has faced, and continues to face, major obstacles. Perhaps most significant of these is the misconception of school administrators and teachers that PE classes compete with academic curricular offerings and negatively influence academic performance. On the contrary, several studies have shown that school-based PE not only did not harm academic performance but also is effective in increasing levels of physical activity and improving physical fitness. Other studies have demonstrated that children who are regularly physically active are less likely to gain weight and also improve academic performance.

18.4   HEALTH CARE SERVICE POLICIES

The National Commission for Quality Assurance (NCQA) for the past decade has approved the Health care Effectiveness Data Information Set (HEDIS) to measure health plan performance [15]. The metrics include the measurement of physical activity and BMI as "vital signs" among adults, children, and adolescents. In addition, nutrition, physical activity assessment, and counseling for all adults, children, and adolescents were also recommended. Most US health plans use HEDIS measures to assess provider performance associated with patient care and services and report to providers and purchasers of health plans and consumers on the quality of health care throughout the nation.

The Patient Protection and Affordable Care Act (also known as the Affordable Care Act; ACC) of 2010 attempted to overhaul the US delivery system to be more proactive in the area of prevention. One element of the ACA was an attempt to impact obesity prevention through the health care delivery system. This involved increased Medicaid payments for preventive care service and managed care for primary care services provided by primary care doctors (family medicine, primary care physicians, general internal medicine, and pediatric medicine) including a 10% bonus payment for primary care physicians in Medicare from 2011 to 2015 [16]. These actions were intended to provide greater incentives for primary care providers to integrate preventive services into their practices. As a practical matter, there has not been a wide adoption of this initiative. However, since obesity represents a very significant financial burden on the health care system and, in particular, is associated with increased risk of a variety of costly conditions, it is only a matter of time until obesity factors into the key area where prevention must take place.

18.5 URBAN DESIGN, LAND USE, AND TRANSPORTATION POLICIES FOR ACTIVE LIVING/HEALTHY EATING

Access to places for physical activity and community-scale environmental infrastructure has been demonstrated to play a positive role in promoting physical activity and active living [17,18]. Open space and outdoor recreational activities provide a place for people to participate in active endeavors. These spaces include parks, green spaces, sports fields, walking and biking trails, covered pools, and playgrounds. A well-developed infrastructure supporting walking is an important element of the built environment and has been demonstrated in a number of studies to be associated with increased activity in both adults and children.

Zoning for mixed-use development is one type of community land use policy and practice that allows residential, commercial, institutional, and other uses to be located in close proximity to one another. This represents a good community-wide strategy for helping to increase physical activity and thereby lower the likelihood of weight gain and obesity.

18.6 CONCLUSIONS

A number of studies have shown that national, state, and local initiatives can affect energy balance behaviors through strategies to increase active living and healthy eating. These include school-based access to healthy eating and active living as well as aspects of the built environment. Comprehensive policy strategies can do considerable good to support health care providers and help prevent weight gain and the associated adverse outcomes of overweight and obesity. These policies also can create an environment where active living and healthy eating are considered to be the usual standards rather than unusual. These represent cost-effective strategies for reducing the risk of weight gain and obesity.

CLINICAL APPLICATIONS

- Clinicians should become involved in community strategies to help lower the risk of overweight and obesity.
- Such strategies include leadership in the areas of healthy eating and increased physical activity.
- Such strategies should include interest in the built environment as well as school siting and practices to encourage children to become more physically active and eat more healthy and nutritious foods.

REFERENCES

1. Hajart A., Weisser S., Wilkerson G., et al. Lifestyle medicine in an era of health care reform, Seven years of healthcare disruption: 2010–2017. In Rippe J.M. (ed.) *Lifestyle Medicine*, 3rd ed. CRC Press, Boca Raton, FL, 2019.

2. Dodson E., Health G. Policy and environmental supports in promoting physical activity and active living. In Rippe J.M. (ed.) *Lifestyle Medicine*, 3rd ed. CRC Press, Boca Raton, FL, 2019.

3. CDC. Recommended community strategies and measurements to prevent obesity in the United States. *MMWR*. 2009; 58(RR-7):1–29.

4. Dietary Guidelines for Americans 2015–2020. https://health.gov/our-work/food-nutrition/2015-2020-dietary-guidelines/guidelines/. Accessed August 31, 2020

5. Penchansky R., Thomas J. The concept of access: Definition, and relationship to consumer satisfaction. *Medical Care*. 1981; 19(2):127–140.

6. Morland K., Wing S., Diez R., et al. Neighborhood characteristics associated with the location of food stores and food service places. *Am J Prev Med*. 2002; 22:23–29.

7. Larson N., Story M., Nelson M.C. Neighborhood environments: disparities in access to healthy foods in the U.S. *Am J Prev Med*. 2008; 36:74–81.

8. Zenk S., Schulz A., Hollis-Neely T., et al. Fruit and vegetable intake in African Americans' income and store characteristics. *Am J Prev Med*. 2005; 29:1–9.

9. Dietz W., Benken D., Hunter A.S. Public health law and the prevention and control of obesity. *Milbank Q*. 2009; 87:215–227.

10. U.S. Department of Health and Human Services. Physical Activity Guidelines for Americans, 2nd edition. Washington, DC: U.S. Department of Health and Human Services, 2018.

11. Saelens B., Sallis J., Frank L. Environmental correlates of walking and cycling: Findings from the transportation, urban design, and planning literatures. *Ann Behav Med*. 2003; 25(2):80–91.

12. Ewing R., Cervero R. Travel and the built environment. *Transp Res Rec*. 2001; 1780:87–114.

13. Ebbeling C., Feldman H., Osganian S., et al. Effects of decreasing sugar-sweetened beverage consumption on body weight in adolescents: A randomized, controlled pilot study. *Pediatrics*. 2006; 117:673–680.

14. National Association for Sport and Physical Education and American Health Association (NASPE). Shape of the nation report: status of physical education in the USA. Reston, VA: National Association for Sport and Physical Education.

15. National Committee for Quality Assurance (NCQA). Performance measures for Wellness and Healthy Promotion Accreditation, 2011. https://www.ncqa.org/wp-content/uploads/2018/08/20180827_PHM_PHM_Resource_Guide.pdf. Accessed August 31, 2020.

16. Henry J. Kaiser Foundation. Summary of new health reform law. https://www.kff.org/health-reform/fact-sheet/summary-of-the-affordable-care-act/. Accessed August 31, 2020.

17. Heath G., Brownson R., Kruger J., et al. The effectiveness of urban design and land use and transport policies and practices to increase physical activity: A systematic review. *J Phys Act Health*. 2006; 3(Suppl 1):S55–S76.

18. Kahn E., Ramsey L., Brownson R., et al. The effectiveness of interventions to increase physical activity. A systematic review. *Am J Prev Med*. 2002; 22(4 Suppl):73–107.

19 Future Directions in Obesity and Weight Management

James M. Rippe, MD
Rippe Lifestyle Institute
University of Massachusetts Medical School

CONTENTS

DOI: 10.1201/9781003099116-22

19.1 INTRODUCTION

The world is in the midst of a pandemic of obesity. It has been estimated that there are over 2.1 billion people with obesity in the world [1]. Obesity is one of the leading preventable causes of death and disease globally, yet the rates of obesity around the globe continue to increase. It has been estimated by the National Institute of Health (NIH) that there are over 300,000 preventable deaths every year in the United States as a result of overweight or obesity [2]. This makes obesity the second leading cause of preventable deaths in the United States behind only cigarette smoking and tobacco exposure.

Moreover, obesity has continued to rise around the world over the past four decades. Overweight and obesity affect not only the developed world but also increasingly the developing world [3]. In addition, treating obesity and its comorbidities is extremely costly. It has been estimated that the global economic impact for obesity alone is approximately $2.1 trillion per year [4].

For the last four decades, experts in public health and medicine have been calling attention to the health threat of the rising pandemic of obesity. Despite considerable interest in the public health community on reducing obesity, progress has fallen well short of expectations.

At the same time, understandings about the biological and behavioral drivers of obesity have continued to advance although there is still incomplete knowledge about the complete pathophysiology of obesity. An increasing number of treatment options have also become available (see also Chapters 8 and 9) and health care providers are increasingly acquiring skills to manage obesity.

Given the prevalence of obesity and its significant adverse health consequences, it is important that we continue to define ways of enhancing both our knowledge and practical application of ways to combat this pandemic.

This will require a combination of new thinking as well as how technologies and a deep commitment on the part of both individual clinicians and also public health professionals if we are going to make headway on this pandemic.

19.2 LIFESTYLE MEDICINE AND THE OBESITY EPIDEMIC

In many ways, obesity represents the quintessential lifestyle condition [5]. While many underlying etiologies contribute to obesity, they all funnel through an imbalance between energy consumption and energy expenditure. While there is certainly a genetic component to weight gain and obesity, many of the comorbidities appear to be more closely related to epigenetics which is the study of how daily habits and actions impact how messages in the genome are actually delivered. The science of epigenetics has suggested that many of these changes in how the genetic map is ultimately handled are strongly related to lifestyle decisions and actions.

19.2.1 PHYSICAL ACTIVITY

Physical activity conveys multiple health benefits including being an important component, not only for short-term weight loss, but also long-term maintenance of weight loss. Abundant new evidence is available from the Physical Activity Guidelines for Americans 2018 Scientific Report (PAGA) about the multiple benefits conveyed by regular physical activity [6]. It is hoped that the availability of this information from this authoritative source will help clinicians include physical activity, not only as a central component of weight management but also as a technique for reducing the risk of multiple comorbidities of obesity such as cardiovascular disease (CVD), type 2 diabetes (T2DM), some cancers, metabolic syndrome (MetS), osteoarthritis, and many other chronic conditions.

19.2.2 NUTRITION

Sound nutritional practices are a critically important component of not only weight maintenance, but also weight loss, in individuals with obesity or who are overweight. There has been increased consumption of energy-dense foods in the United States over the past 40 years. There has also been a recent emphasis on plant-based dieting in the United States. Plant-based dieting has the potential to help in the control of weight and is an important component of weight loss. Plant-based diets are, by their very nature, nutrient dense and not energy dense (See also Chapter 6).

19.2.3 BEHAVIORAL APPROACHES TO WEIGHT MANAGEMENT

Many of the lifestyle modalities which are important for maintenance of a healthy weight and also weight loss for individuals with obesity or who are overweight involve changing behaviors. In this area, there are multiple frameworks that have been shown to be valuable for weight loss or maintenance of a healthy weight (See also Chapter 7). In the future, it is hoped that clinicians will become knowledgeable about the various potential behavior frameworks that have been demonstrated to help in weight maintenance.

19.2.4 MOTIVATIONAL INTERVIEWING

Motivational interviewing (MI) has been demonstrated to be an effective modality in multiple chronic conditions including obesity management. This technique involves clinicians establishing an open-ended relationship with patients where the patient's needs, wants, and desires take center stage [7]. This is in contrast to the prevalent medical model where the physician is seen as an expert and dispenses advice. MI has the potential for effective utilization in individuals with obesity or who are overweight. We hope that more clinicians will become knowledgeable about this technique in the future.

19.2.5 POSITIVE PSYCHOLOGY

There has been recent interest and a large number of publications in the area of positive psychology [8]. This technique, which emphasizes individual patient's strengths, has potential to positively impact on maintenance of a healthy weight, weight loss, and reduction in obesity. Multiple resources are available to describe this technique.

19.2.6   COACHING

Significant growth has occurred in the past decade in the profession of coaching. Coaches are trained to help guide patients through behavior change and help patients overcome barriers [9]. Coaches can supplement work that clinicians perform in the area of weight management.

19.2.7   STRESS REDUCTION

In the modern, fast-paced world there is an enormous need for stress reduction. Oftentimes, people compensate for stress in their lives by overeating. There is also an established link between stress and eating energy-dense foods. ("Comfort" foods actually often live up to their name!) There are multiple techniques available for stress reduction and these should be a component that lifestyle medicine practitioners utilize in the treatment of overweight and obesity [10].

19.2.8   SLEEP

The topic of the health impact of sleep has recently assumed significant interest in the research community [11]. Lifestyle medicine practitioners should discuss sleep patterns with all overweight or obese individuals. Inadequate amounts of sleep have been clearly correlated with weight gain and obesity. Sleep will undoubtedly become an important obesity research topic in the future.

19.3   NEW PARADIGMS FOR PRACTICING MEDICINE

The Covid-19 pandemic in the United States and around the world has caused clinicians to rethink the way that we practice medicine. There has been a very significant increase in telemedicine. This type of technology offers an opportunity for clinicians to efficiently discuss lifestyle medicine issues including weight management and obesity. Telemedicine encounters may also make discussing weight more comfortable and acceptable to many overweight or obese patients.

19.4   REMOVING BARRIERS TO BETTER OUTCOMES

Despite considerable interest in and increased knowledge from a variety of aspects concerning weight gain and obesity, little progress has been made in slowing down the pandemic. There may be some opportunities to improve existing protocols but this will require removing systemic barriers such as entrenched bias and stigma, as well as inadequate clinical resources for delivering effective obesity care and payment systems that presently favor treating the complications of obesity rather than preventing those complications.

19.4.1   ENTRENCHED BIAS AND STIGMA

There is considerable evidence of bias and stigma concerning individuals with obesity [12]. This bias typically begins in childhood [13,14]. Obesity awareness campaigns may even promote this stigma without improving access to clinically effective care [15]. Both the American Medical Association (AMA) [16] and the American Academy of Pediatrics (AAP) [17] have formally resolved to work toward reducing the harm of weight bias in pediatric, adolescent, and adult medicine. In addition, popular media has increasingly drawn attention to this problem which has been characterized as "fat shaming" in an attempt to make such stigma unacceptable in popular culture [18]. Supporting body positivity has the potential to improve the quality of life of people affected by obesity.

19.4.2 INADEQUATE RESOURCES FOR OBESITY CARE

In 2013, the American Medical Association characterized obesity as a "disease" [18]. Unfortunately, despite this recognition, clinical practice patterns do not affect that perception. For example, approximately 5 million children have severe obesity in the United States, yet fewer than 50 centers have Class 3 programs for pediatric obesity care [19]. Most health care providers have relatively good training for delivering evidence-based obesity care but do not express high confidence in providing such care. There are, however, some reasons for optimism in this area. The American Board of Obesity Medicine has reported that over 2,000 physicians have now become Board certified in obesity medicine which makes it one of the fastest-growing fields in medical care [20]. Furthermore, there is a real opportunity for practitioners in lifestyle medicine to acquire the skills necessary to deliver high-quality obesity treatment.

19.4.3 PAYMENT SYSTEMS FAVOR TREATING OBESITY COMPLICATIONS RATHER THAN OBESITY

Payment systems typically deny or severely restrict coverage for obesity yet fully cover treatment for most of its complications. These complications include CVD, T2DM, many forms of cancer, arthritis, liver disease, and many others. Direct medical costs of obesity have been estimated at $149 million. It has been estimated that the total US economic burden for obesity-related complications is $1.4 trillion dollars [21].

The Affordable Care Act was intended to increase insurance coverage for obesity treatment. Many insurance plans, however, still do not cover obesity treatment [22]. Pharmacotherapy for obesity is very limited. One study found that only 11% of policies in only nine states covered anti-obesity drugs [23]. Bariatric surgery coverage is relatively more common than lifestyle therapy or pharmacotherapy. For example, since 2006, Medicare has covered this form of obesity care [24]. Unfortunately, relatively few patients seek clinical care for obesity perhaps because they may have an internalized stigma which may lead many of these individuals to assume that obesity is a self-inflicted condition that they must bear full responsibility for resolving.

Finding ways to improve access to well-established and effective obesity care represents an untapped opportunity for improved outcomes in the population that is affected by this condition.

19.5   MORE EFFECTIVE PUBLIC HEALTH
STRATEGIES IN THE FUTURE

Much of the focus in the area of obesity has been focused on prevention yet, the prevalence of obesity in both childhood and adults has grown considerably over the past 40 years. Thus, it is important to focus on effective ways to both prevent and treat obesity.

19.5.1   A NARROW FOCUS ON FOOD POLICY

It is important to think about a variety of factors that impact obesity. This would include not only various aspects of nutrition including food policy [25], but also an emphasis on physical activity which would also promote better health in a variety of different ways. While the application of physical activity and better nutrition has not been highly successful in the past, a more sophisticated approach to these modalities through lifestyle medicine could yield important and cost-effective ways of preventing and treating obesity.

19.5.2   ACCOUNTING FOR COMPLEX SYSTEMS DRIVING OBESITY

The pandemic of obesity should be viewed as a product of complex systems that interact with each other, often in unpredictable ways [26]. This will require input from multiple disciplines and also collaboration between various industry, academic, government, and nonprofit organizations. Better results that have been achieved in the past will only come from an approach that is more grounded in evidence from multiple different disciplines.

19.6   NEW TECHNOLOGIES

A wide range of new technologies are available that are beginning to impact a variety of aspects of lifestyle. For example, wearable technologies have enhanced the likelihood that individuals can monitor physiologic responses to physical activity. Programs that are based on the Internet and/or utilize smartphone technologies [27] may also help people who are trying to lose weight achieve not only information but also a broader sense of community [27]. In the future, we are likely to see more commercial obesity treatment programs utilize these types of technologies. It will be important for the medical community to also embrace these new technologies in order to play an active and important role in obesity treatment.

19.7   NEW VISIONS FOR HEALTH

While the Covid-19 pandemic has been a source of enormous pain, discomfort, and fear for people around the world, there may be a silver lining in this whole tragedy. Perhaps people will utilize this opportunity to consider new ways of thinking about their health. While this is speculation, there is a history of individuals rising to meet tragedies. One individual who has written persuasively about how terrible situations such as the Holocaust can bring about new patterns of thinking is Viktor Frankl who wrote that "we don't get to choose our difficulties, but we do have the freedom to select our responses" [28]. He argued that meaning comes from three things: the work we offer in times of crisis, the love we give, and our ability to display courage in the place of suffering.

While obesity does not carry the same acute danger as COVID-19, it certainly carries an enormous long-term danger with over 2 billion people suffering from this condition and also increasing their risk of various comorbidities. Perhaps as individuals rise to meet the challenge of Covid-19, there will also be an impetus to think in broader terms about what each of us does on a daily basis to enhance our health. This could offer some hope for addressing the pandemic of obesity.

19.8 RESEARCH PRIORITIES

One area which has potential to help combat the obesity epidemic is the advances that are occurring in pharmacotherapy and other aspects of medicine such as "precision medicine".

19.8.1 ADVANCES IN PHARMACOTHERAPY

Before 2013, there had not been much innovation in pharmacotherapy for obesity. In 1996, Dexfenfluramine was approved which was the first new weight loss medicine the FDA had approved in years. However, in 1997, it was withdrawn from the market after reports of unacceptably high risk of valvular heart disease [28]. Two other prescription drugs were approved by the FDA shortly thereafter – Sibutramine and Orlistat; however, both had disappointing results in the market. Sibutramine was withdrawn in 2010 [29].

The FDA also responded by raising safety thresholds for approving new drugs targeted for weight loss. The first drug that fell into this regulatory problem was Rimonabant which had been approved in Europe but was not approved in the United States. The FDA finally began approving obesity drugs again in 2013 [30] A variety of new drugs are now available with a potential benefit for improving weight loss. (These are discussed in more detail in Chapter 8.)

19.8.2 PRECISION MEDICINE

Given that there is a genetic component to obesity, there is some potential to explain an individual's susceptibility to obesity [31]. Much of this depends on genetic testing which may potentially lead to what has been called "precision medicine" [32,33].

19.8.3 ATTENTION TO LONG-TERM OUTCOMES

A key to lowering the health risk of obesity is finding long-term solutions. Several areas where there is good evidence are CVD and T2DM. Some studies have suggested a reduction of risk of these comorbidities following weight loss. It is anticipated that there will be more focus on long-term outcomes moving forward.

19.8.4 TRANSLATIONAL SCIENCE

It is important that research findings in obesity become translated into clinical practice. Of particular area of interest is how the well-established benefits of physical activity and lower consumption of high-calorie foods may benefit lowering the risk of obesity. Emerging science in the areas of stress reduction and sleep will also be very important if they can be adequately translated to the public [34].

19.9 SUMMARY/CONCLUSIONS

While the pandemic of obesity has continued to increase over the past four decades, there is reason to believe that the future will hold some opportunities to lower this pandemic on the enormous human and economic toll that it has taken.

CLINICAL APPLICATIONS

* It is important for lifestyle medicine clinicians to evaluate every patient for weight gain and obesity.
* Application of key areas of lifestyle medicine including regular physical activity, proper nutrition, adequate sleep, and stress reduction can help ameliorate this worldwide pandemic.
* Future lifestyle therapies as well as advances in technologies, genetics, and pharmacologic approaches all hold considerable promise for the future.

REFERENCES

1. Hales C., Carroll M., Fryar C., et al. Prevalence of obesity among adults and youth: United States, 2015–2016. US Department of Health and Human Services, Centers for Disease Control and Prevention, National Center for Health Statistics; Oct 2017.
2. Flegal K., Williamson D., Pamuk E., et al. Estimating deaths attributable to obesity in the United States. *Am J Public Health*. 2004; 94(9):1486–9.
3. The GBD 2015 Obesity Collaborators. Health effects of overweight and obesity in 195 countries over 25 years. *N Engl J Med*. 2017; 377(1):13–27.
4. Day R., Jitnarin N., Vidoni M. et al. Epidemiology of adult obesity. In Rippe J.M. (ed.) *Lifestyle Medicine*, 3rd ed. CRC Press, Boca Raton, FL, 2019.
5. Rippe J.M. Lifestyle medicine: The health promoting power of daily habits and practices. Am *J Lifestyle Med*. 2018; 13:6.
6. 2018 Physical Activity Guidelines for Americans. Washington, DC. US Department of Health and Human Services, 2018. https://health.gov/sites/default/files/2019-09/Physical_Activity_Guidelines_2nd_edition.pdf. Accessed August 28, 2020.
7. Fifield P., Suzuki J., Minski S. et al. Motivational interviewing and lifestyle change. In Rippe J.M. (ed.) *Lifestyle Medicine*, 3rd ed. CRC Press, Boca Raton, FL, 2019.
8. Carson S., Cook A., Peabody S., et al. The impact of positive psychology on behavioral change and healthy lifestyle choices. In Rippe J.M. (ed.) *Lifestyle Medicine*, 3rd ed. CRC Press, Boca Raton, FL, 2019.
9. International Coaching Federation. https://coachfederation.org/. Accessed August 28, 2020.
10. Nedley N., Ramirez F. Emotional health and stress reduction. In Rippe J.M. (ed.) *Lifestyle Medicine*. 3rd ed. CRC Press, Boca Raton, FL, 2019.

11. 2018 Physical Activity Guidelines for Americans. Washington, DC. US Department of Health and Human Services, 2018. Part F. Chapter 3. Brain Health. https://health.gov/sites/default/files/2019-09/09_F-3_Brain_Health.pdf. Accessed August 28, 2020.

12. Puhl R., Heuer C. Obesity stigma: Important considerations for public health. *Am J Public Health*. 2010; 100(6):1019–28.

13. de la Haye K., Dijkstra J., Lubbers M., et al. The dual role of friendship and antipathy relations in the marginalization of overweight children in their peer networks: The TRAILS Study. *PloS One*. 2017; 12(6):e0178130.

14. Skinner A., Payne K., Perrin A., et al. Implicit weight bias in children age 9 to 11 years. *Pediatrics*. 2017; 140(1):e20163936.

15. Puhl R., King K. Weight discrimination and bullying. *Best Pract Res Clin Endocrinol Metab*. 2013; 27(2):117–27.

16. AMA Destigmatize Obesity Resolution [Internet]. Obesity Medicine Association, 2017. https://obesitymedicine.org/ama-destigmatize-obesity-resolution. Accessed August 28, 2020.

17. Pont S., Puhl R., Cook S., et al. Stigma experienced by children and adolescents with obesity. *Pediatrics*. 2017:e20173034.

18. Bergland C. Sizeism Is Harming Too Many of Us: Fat Shaming Must Stop [Internet]. Psychology Today. Sussex Publishers, 2017 [cited Feb. 12, 2018]. https://www.psychologytoday.com/blog/the-athletes-way/201708/sizeism-is-harming-too-many-us-fat-shaming-must-stop.

19. Kyle T. Childhood Obesity Treatment Programs: A Few to Serve Many. ConscienHealth, 2018. https://conscienhealth.org/2018/09/why-is-respectful-care-for-childhood-obesity-remarkable/. Accessed August 28, 2020.

20. American Board of Obesity Medicine Surpasses 2,000 Diplomates. Business Wire. American Board of Obesity Medicine, 2017. https://www.businesswire.com/news/home/20170216005152/en/American-Board-Obesity-Medicine-Surpasses-2000-Diplomates. Accessed August 28, 2020.

21. Waters H, DeVol R. Weighing down America: The health and economic impact of obesity. Milken Institute Center for Public Health. November 2016. www.milkeninstitute.org. Accessed June 7, 2021

22. Wilson E., Kyle T., Nadglowski J., et al. Obesity coverage gap: consumers perceive low coverage for obesity treatments even when workplace wellness programs target BMI. *Obesity*. 2017; 25(2):370–7.

23. Gomez G., Stanford F.C. US health policy and prescription drug coverage of FDA-approved medications for the treatment of obesity. *Int J Obes (Lond)*. 2018; 42(3):495–500.

24. Batsis J., Bynum J. Uptake of the centers for Medicare and Medicaid obesity benefit: 2012–2013. *Obesity*. 2016; 24(9):1983–8.

25. Roberto C., Swinburn B., Hawkes C., et al. Patchy progress on obesity prevention: Emerging examples, entrenched barriers, and new thinking. *The Lancet*. 2015; 385(9985):2400–9.

26. Vandenbroeck I., Goossens J., Clemens M. Building the obesity system map. Foresight Tackling Obesities: Future Choices. https://assets.publishing.service.gov.uk/government/uploads/system/uploads/attachment_data/file/295154/07-1179-obesity-building-system-map.pdf. Accessed August 28, 2020.

27. 2018 Physical Activity Guidelines for Americans. Washington, DC. US Department of Health and Human Services, 2018. Part F. Chapter 11. Promoting Regular Physical Activity. https://health.gov/sites/default/files/2019-09/17_F-11_Promoting_Regular_Physical_Activity.pdf. Accessed August 28, 2020.

28. Elliot W., Chan J. Fenfluramine and Dexfenfluramine Withdrawn from Market. AHC Media. 1997. https://www.reliasmedia.com/articles/48147-fenfluramine-and-dexfenfluramine-withdrawn-from-market. Accessed August 28, 2020.

29. In Brief: Sibutramine (Meridia) Withdrawn]. The Medical Letter on Drugs and Therapeutics. Medical Letter, Inc.; 2010. https://secure.medicalletter.org/w1350d.
30. Kyle T. Favoring Innovation in Obesity. ConscienHealth. 2014. http://conscienhealth.org/2014/09/favoring-innovation-in-obesity/. Accessed August 28, 2020.
31. Musani S., Erickson S., Allison D.B. Obesity: Still highly heritable after all these years. *Am J Clin Nutr.* 2008; 87(2):275.
32. Locke A., Kahali B., Berndt S., et al. Genetic studies of body mass index yield new insights for obesity biology. *Nature.* 2015; 518(7538):197.
33. Yanovski S., Yanovski J. Toward precision approaches for the prevention and treatment of obesity. *JAMA.* 2018; 319(3):223–4.
34. Dietz W., Solomon L., Pronk N., et al. An integrated framework for the prevention and treatment of obesity and its related chronic diseases. *Health Aff.* 2015; 34(9):1456–63.

Index

Note: **Bold** page numbers refer to tables and *italic* page numbers refer to figures.

For Product Safety Concerns and Information please contact our EU
representative GPSR@taylorandfrancis.com
Taylor & Francis Verlag GmbH, Kaufingerstraße 24, 80331 München, Germany

www.ingramcontent.com/pod-product-compliance
Ingram Content Group UK Ltd.
Pitfield, Milton Keynes, MK11 3LW, UK
UKHW021441080625
459435UK00011B/332